Cognitive Screening and Testing Tools

Computerized Cognitive Assessment Products

Neurocognitive Screening for ADHD, Memory Loss, Alzheimer's, Dementia, Traumatic Brain Injury

2013 Edition

ISBN: 0615836011
ISBN-13: 978-0615836010 (MyBrainTest)

About MyBrainTest

MyBrainTest.org is a market research and advisory service for the cognitive health assessment and testing market, and the larger neurodiagnostic industry. We provide an independent source of information on brain health screening tests for Alzheimer's, dementia, and brain injuries such as sports concussions.

Globally, we are at the front edge of a rising wave of dementia impairment as the population ages, and this wave of millions will severely strain national health care systems. Early intervention with baseline memory screening and testing will be key to managing exploding health care costs associated with Alzheimer's disease and other types of dementia.

MyBrainTest
1010 University Avenue
Suite 1570
San Diego, California 92103
info@mybraintest.org
www.mybraintest.org

Report Contents

Report Contents (cont)

EXECUTIVE SUMMARY

Since our last report in 2011, the market for computerized cognitive assessment, screening and testing has continued to expand. Key drivers for this market and growing technology product base include:

An Aging Global Population. There **are more than 500 million people** alive in the world today who are older than age 65. Dementia rates begin to rise sharply in this population group after age 75. Having reliable, easy to use tools to screen for memory and cognitive impairment will become increasingly important.

Increased Awareness of Cognitive Health Issues. Media stories have highlighted the negative long term health consequences of multiple concussions in team sports. Parents, schools, and physicians require tools to screen and treat children with Autism Spectrum Disorder or ADHD (which many times overlap.) Standardized cognitive screening tools will help support diagnostic certainty and treatment.

Rapid Advances in Technology Platforms. Tablet devices with secure wireless access to "big data" psychometric norms and reports are augmenting, and in some cases replacing large, stationary desktop PC platforms. Portable cognitive screening can begin to move into the field and be rapidly configured in primary care/general practice settings.

RISING DEMENTIA RATES ARE A GLOBAL HEALTH TREND

A positive aspect of rising living standards in most of the world has been a significant improvement in average worldwide life expectancies, increasing from 52 years in 1960 to 69 years in 2009. Regional differences are even more striking -- the average life expectancy for a person living in North America has risen from 70 years in 1960 to 78 years in 2009, while the life expectancy in East Asia & Pacific countries as a group has grown from 47 years to 73 years during this same period. [(1)]

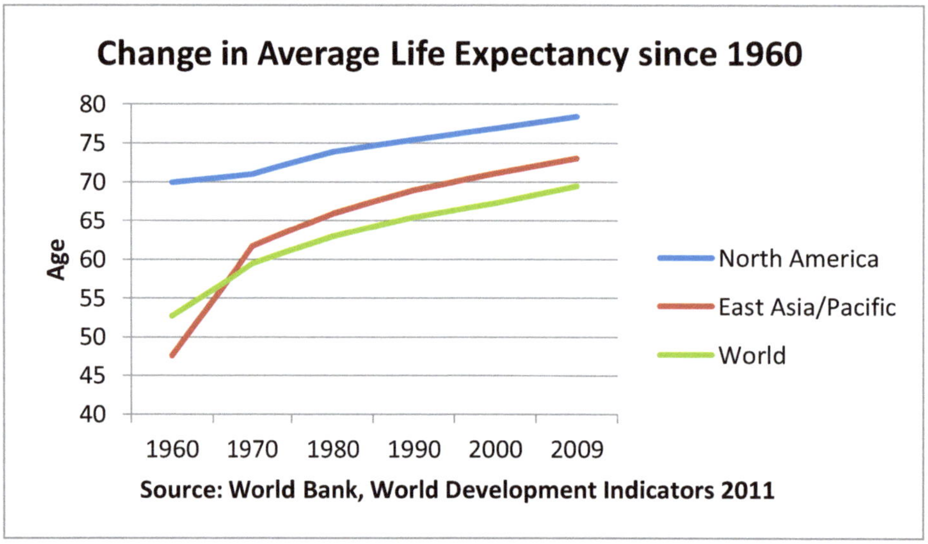

DEMENTIA SUBTYPES

Dementia is an age related, progressive neurocognitive disorder. Dementia encompasses several subtypes, including Alzheimer's disease (about 70% of all cases), vascular dementia, dementia with Lewy bodies, and frontotemporal dementia. Mixed dementia, such as Alzheimer's with vascular dementia, is also a common subtype.

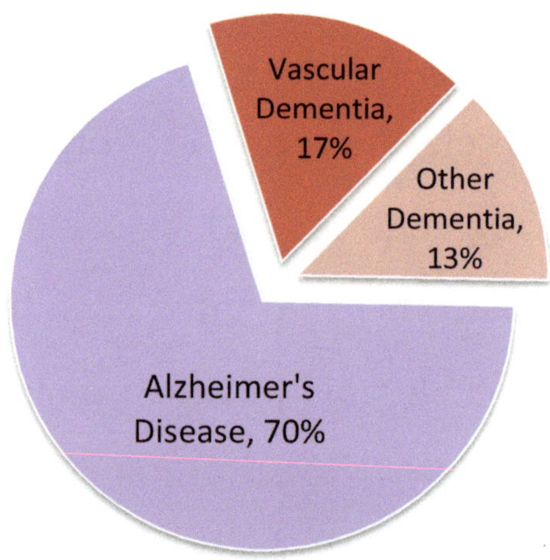

Plassman, et al, Prevalence of Dementia in the United States, Neuroepidimiology 2007, 29: 125-132

ESTIMATED DEMENTIA PREVALENCE RATES

The RAND Corporation and American Academy of Neurology (AAN) have conducted national dementia prevalence studies in the past year.[2,3] The results from these studies show that the rate of dementia increases significantly in age groups of 75 and older:

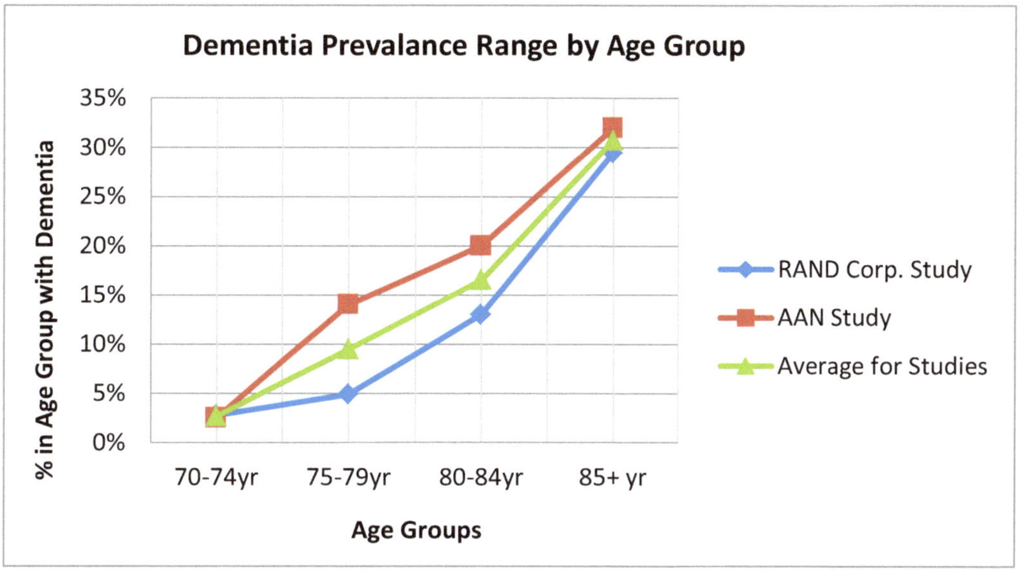

Over 35 million people are living with dementia worldwide today, and this number is projected to increase to 66 million in 2030 and 115 million by 2050.[4] The rapid rise in global dementia cases over the next 30-40 years will present a series of challenges for health care providers, governments, and families, ranging from overburdened health care systems, to the need for public awareness and education about dementia signs and symptoms. Another important part is the need for standardized dementia screening guidelines.

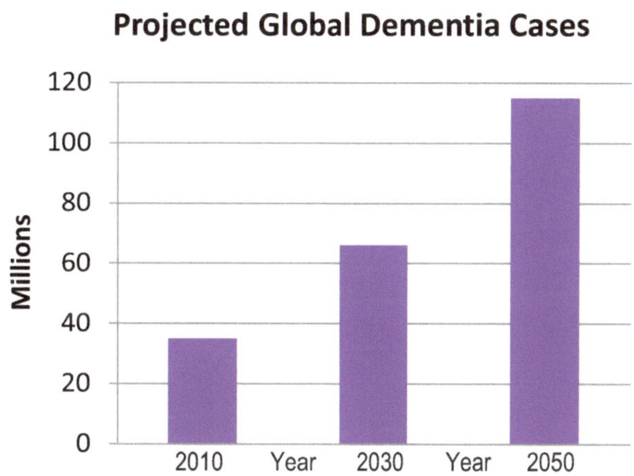

Source: Alzheimer's Disease International Report 2010

MEASURING COGNITIVE HEALTH AT ALL AGES

CONCUSSION AND TRAUMATIC BRAIN INJURY

Every year in the United States, at least **1.7 million** people sustain a traumatic brain injury (TBI) or concussion that is severe enough to require medical evaluation. Sports-related hospital emergency department (ER) admissions total 250,000 per year.[5] American football, soccer, and cycling are the top activities that bring children and teenagers to the ER for concussion and brain injury symptoms.

High risk occupations such as military service also contribute to TBI rates. Several studies have indicated TBI rates of around 10%-20% from the 2001-2009 Iraq & Afghanistan deployments, or about 150K to 300K service members. [6] Problems with memory, focus, attention, balance and coordination are very common with blast related TBI.

A serious lack of TBI assessment tools is now beginning to be addressed by products like the Defense Automated Neurobehavioral Assessment (DANA) system and BrainFx.

AUSTISM SPECTRUM DISORDER AND ADHD

In May 2013, U.S. Centers for Disease Control (CDC) published a comprehensive summary of the epidemiology of childhood brain disorders, including Autism Spectrum Disorder, and Attention-deficit/hyperactivity disorder (ADHD). [7] Key findings from the study include:

- Over **5 million** children aged 3-17 in the US have been diagnosed with ADHD. Boys are more than twice as likely as girls to receive an ADHD diagnosis.
- Nearly **1 million** children aged 3-17 in the US have been diagnosed with Autism Spectrum Disorder (ASD). The male predominance rate of ASD is 3.5 to 4.5 times higher than the female ASD rate.

Standardized cognitive screening tools for ASD and ADHD can help support diagnostic certainty and inform treatment options.

TECHNOLOGY ADVANCES UNDERPIN PERSONALIZED COGNITIVE HEALTH MARKERS

A significant advantage of computerized cognitive screening is the ability to create a baseline cognitive performance test, with annual re-tests, to establish a patient's cognitive health history. Below is an illustrative example of routine memory testing:

Memory Testing - Annual Cognitive Screening

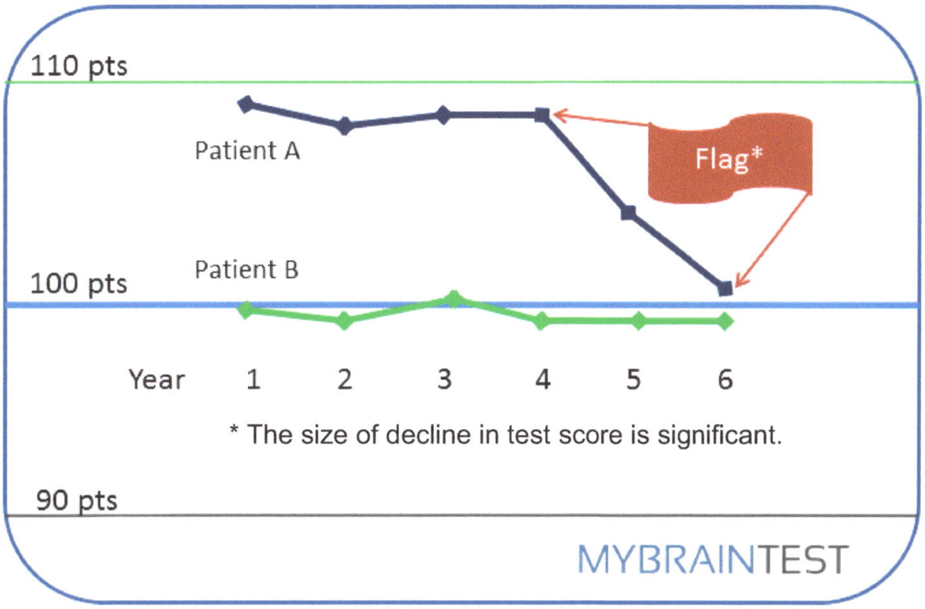

Notice the large drop in Patient A's test scores in years 4 thru 6. This performance drop would likely be a significant "flag" for the reviewing clinician, resulting in more detailed diagnostic tests to determine the cause of this sharp drop in Patient A's memory performance. However, the best way for Patient A's physicians to know about this cognitive health problem is by being able to review the history of Patient A's cognitive screening results, seeing the sharp drop in recent memory scores.

The potential for routine, large scale population screenings are being driven by preventive health initiatives like the Medicare Annual Wellness Visit (AWV), which includes "detection of any cognitive impairment." The AWV is available to over 60 million Medicare members.

ABOUT THE REST OF THIS REPORT

The remainder this report contain detailed information on computerized cognitive testing tools, including **cognitive domains tested, total testing time, and supported technology platforms**. Test report samples from many of these products are also included.

Companies and organizations listed in this computerized cognitive testing guide

- BrainFx
- Brain Resource
- BrainTrain Inc
- Cambridge Cognition
- CNS Vital Signs
- CogState
- HeadMinder
- imPACT Applications
- Medical Care Corp
- Medinteract
- NeuroTrax
- Psychology Software Tools
- Screen Inc.
- US Department of Defense

Physician Use Case examples for cognitive screening begin on page 63.

We welcome questions, comments, and suggestions on how to improve this report. Send an email to info@mybraintest.org

PRODUCT SUMMARY TABLES

PRIMARY USE MATRIX

TEST ADMINISTRATION METHODS

SUPPORTED TECHNOLOGY PLATFORMS

Primary Use Matrix – Computerized Cognitive Tests

Test Name	Neurodegenerative Disorders Screening for Neurodegenerative Disorders (episodic memory loss, MCI, Alzheimer's, other dementias)	Concussion and TBI Screening for concussion and traumatic brain injury (TBI) symptoms	Neuropsychiatric Disorders Screening for Neuropsychiatric Disorders (ADHD, depression, schizophrenia, etc)
BrainFx (p. 15)		●	
CAMCI (p. 56)	●		
CANS-MCI (p. 59)	●		
CANTABmobile (p. 23)	●		
CNS Vital Signs (p. 25)	●	Secondary use	Secondary use
COGNIGRAM (p. 31)	●		
COGselftest (p.44)	●		
CSI (p. 32)	●	Secondary use	Secondary use
DANA (p. 62)		●	
imPACT (p. 35)		●	
IVA+ Plus (p. 20)			●
MCI Screen (p. 42)	●		
MindStreams (p.48)	●	Secondary use	Secondary use
WebNeuro (p. 18)			●

Computerized Cognitive Test Methods and Supported Platforms

	Test Administration Methods			Supported Platforms		
Test Name	Computer admin (with clinician or staff supervision)	Human administered - oral or paper test	Test results are computer scored	Test is accessed by web browser	Test is a Tablet device installed app.	Test is on a PC installed app.
BrainFx (p. 15)	●		●		●	
CAMCI (p. 56)	●		●		●	
CANS-MCI (p. 59)	●		●			●
CANTABmobile (p. 23)	●		●		●	
CNS Vital Signs (p. 25)	●		●			●
COGNIGRAM (p. 31)	●		●		●	
COGselftest (p.44)	●		●	●		
CSI (p. 32)	●		●			●
DANA (p. 62)	●		●		●	
imPACT (p. 35)	●		●			●
IVA+ Plus (p. 20)	●		●			●
MCI Screen (p. 42)		●	●	●		
MindStreams (p.48)	●		●			●
WebNeuro (p. 18)	●		●			●

COMPANY SURVEY SECTION

COGNITIVE TEST PRODUCT DETAIL

TEST REPORT SAMPLES

COMPANY	**BRAINFX, INC.**
LOCATION	Markham, Ontario, Canada
WEBSITE	www.brainfx.com
COGNITIVE TEST PRODUCT	BrainFx 360, a neurofunctional assessment system
TEST FEATURES	
TESTING TIME	60-90 minutes
TESTING PLATFORM	Android Tablet (standard issue) + Web Portal (web browser). Internet connection required.
CAN BE ADMINISTERED BY OFFICE STAFF?	To be administered by regulated health professionals or their supervised support personnel. Both need to complete the BrainFx Administrator certification which is accessible online.
COGNITIVE DOMAINS TESTED	Attention - sustained, selective, to detail, divided Memory - immediate, working, delayed, prospective Temporal (time) awareness Sequencing - simple, complex Problem solving - simple, complex Mental flexibility Abstract Reasoning - categorization, big picture Communication - comprehension, written, verbal Judgment for safety, Foresight for safety Emotion recognition Route Finding Comprehension & Inferences Executive Functioning Information Processing Speed Performance with and without distraction
ADDITIONAL TEST ITEMS	Visual neglect- acuity, perception Hearing - to frequency, to side Fine Motor Function, Static balance Fatigue, Pain, Anxiety scales Self-report questionnaires include: Medical history, Sleep, Nutrition, Activities of Daily Life (ADL) participation and satisfaction Mood, behavior, social symptom checklists

COMPANY	BRAINFX, INC. (CONT)
TEST PRIMARILY USED FOR DETECTION OF:	Complex Traumatic Brain Injury (TBI) Symptoms
TEST VALIDITY AND REFERENCES	See Company End Notes Section for Test Validation References
TEST REPORT FORMAT	Report includes summary level information and scores on individual subtests. Changes from previous assessments are also noted. See sample next page.
PRICING INFORMATION	Health professional certification (online): $395 $75 per assessment. Volume discounts available.

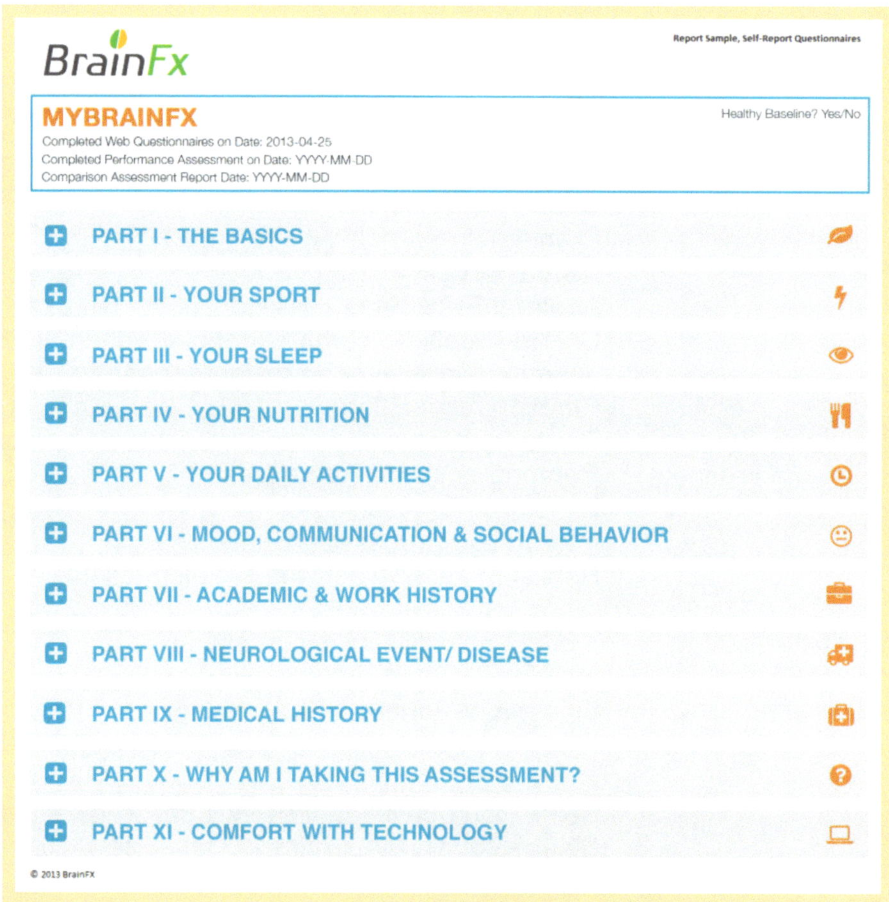

Sample BrainFX Report, Summary of Cognitive Skill Performance

Foundational Skills

64%
Memory – Immediate – For Auditory

51%
Memory – Immediate – For Visual Spatial

93%
Memory – Immediate – For Auditory, Complex, Novel

85%
Memory – Working

78%
Temporal Awareness

Complex Skills

23%
Attention – Divided

65%
Memory – Prospective – Auditory, 2 steps

45%
Memory – Prospective – Visual Cue

78%
Mental Flexibility

60%
Abstract Reasoning

53%
Judgment for safety

27%
Foresight for safety

46%
Comprehension & Humour Inferences

51%
Executive Functioning and Combined Skills

Intermediate Skills

78%
Attention – Selective – To Visual Distraction

56%
Attention – Selective – To Auditory Distraction

45%
Memory – Delayed – For Auditory & Written

29%
Memory – Delayed – For Face and Names (learned under auditory distraction)

36%
Memory – Delayed – For Written and Cued

45%
Problem Solving

56%
Constructive Ability

54%
Route Finding

29%
Sequencing

Social & Behavior Skills

87%
Emotion Recognition

38%
Impulsivity

Pervasive Skills

72%
Information Processing Speed

82%
Endurance

65%
Comprehension & Communication

Company	Brain Resource
Location	Sydney, Australia
Website	www.brainresource.com
Cognitive Test Product	WebNeuro
Test Features	
Testing Time	30-40 minutes
Required Hardware	Internet connection required. PC, Keyboard, mouse.
Can be Administered by Office Staff?	Yes, with training.
Cognitive Domains Tested	Memory, Attention, Language, Executive Function, Emotion Recognition
Test Primarily used for Detection of:	Depression screening, other neuropsychiatric disorders.
Test Validity and References	See Company End Notes Section for Test Validation References
Test Report Format	Consolidated summary report Standard scores for subtests See sample report next page.
Pricing Information	Contact Company

Brain Resource®

Cognition

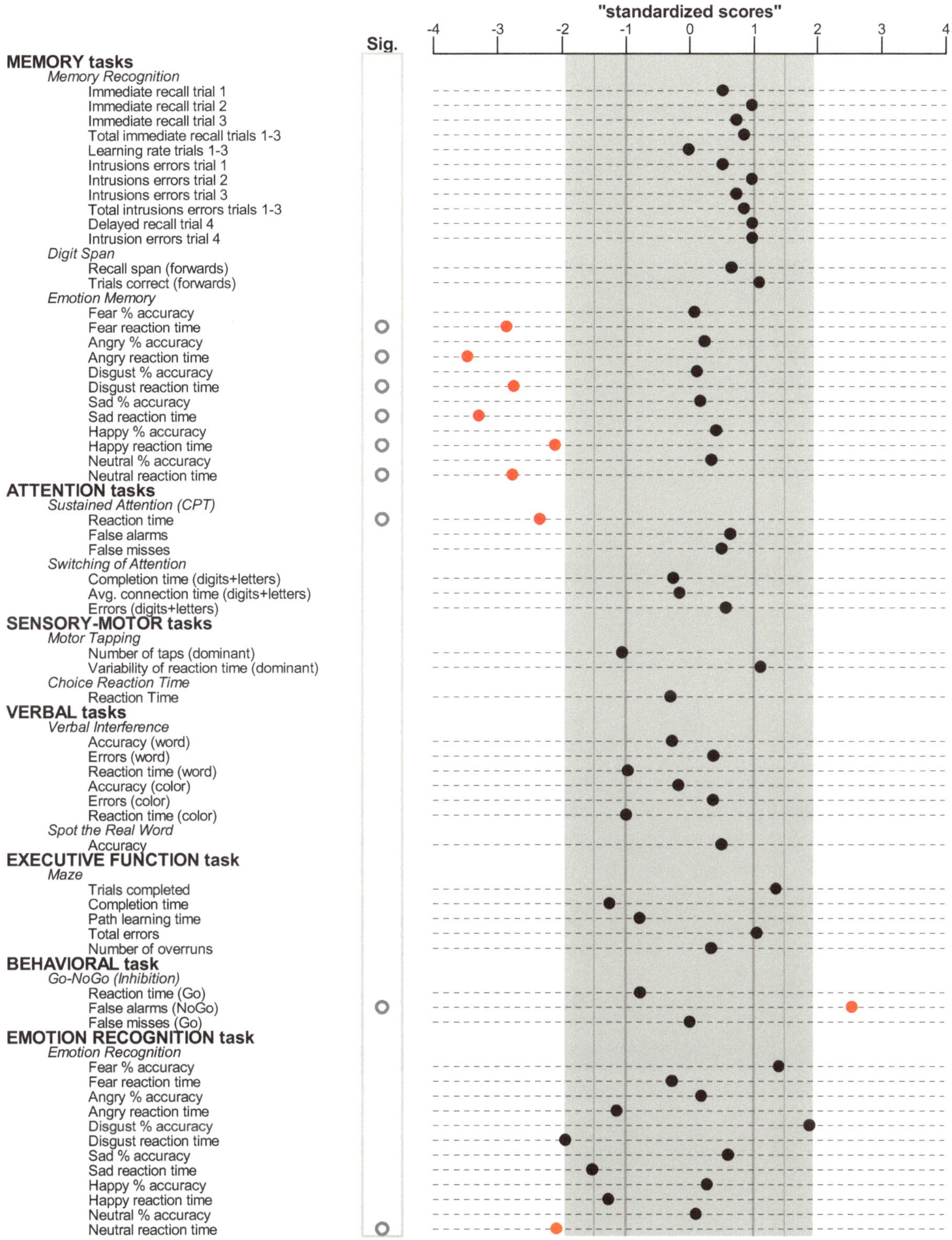

For convenience, the tasks are organized by broad cognitive groupings. The circles on the left indicate statistically significant differences compared with the normal control. The "standardized scores" on the right are normalized for age and gender, which means differences from zero reflect differences from 'average peer' (also known as z-scores). Positive "standardized scores" indicate strengths, negative "standardized scores" indicate potential deficits (Avg = average). "Standardized scores" beyond -2 to +2 are statistically significant. False alarms (respond when should not) = false positive; errors of commission. False misses (not respond when should) = false negatives; errors of omission. Intrusion = words not on the list. Specialist interpretation is required.

COMPANY	BRAINTRAIN, INC.
LOCATION	North Chesterfield, Virginia, USA
WEBSITE	www.braintrain.com
COGNITIVE TEST PRODUCT	IVA+Plus
TEST FEATURES	
TESTING TIME	20 minutes
TESTING PLATFORM	PC, Monitor, Keyboard, External Speakers
CAN BE ADMINISTERED BY OFFICE STAFF?	Yes, by qualified professionals.
COGNITIVE DOMAINS TESTED	Visual and Auditory Attention
TEST PRIMARILY USED FOR DETECTION OF:	ADHD/ADD symptoms
TEST VALIDITY AND REFERENCES	See Company End Notes Section for Test Validation References
TEST REPORT FORMAT	Standard scales See sample report next page.
PRICING INFORMATION	$499 starter kit includes 10 assessments. $1895 for unlimited assessments. $15 per test interpretation (report generation)

IVA+Plus Standard Scales Analysis

Full Scale
Response Control Quotient = 87

Full Scale
Attention Quotient = 99

Auditory RCQ = 77 | Visual RCQ = 102 | Auditory AQ = 99 | Visual AQ = 100

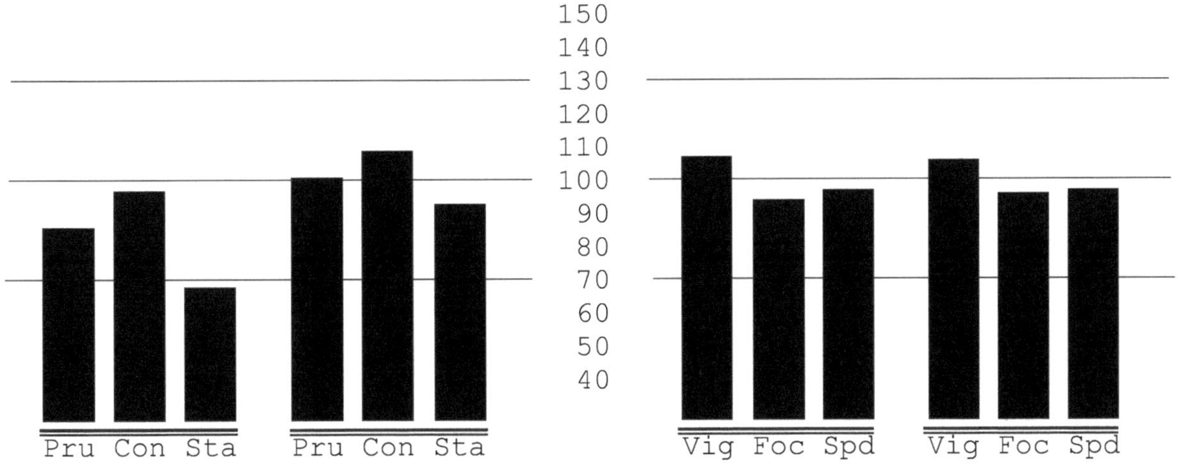

Auditory Response Validity Check = Valid
Visual Response Validity Check = Valid

Fine Motor Hyperactivity: None Mild Mod Sev Ext

PERSONAL INFORMATION

Last Name Train First Name Brain

Social Security # Educational Level 13

Date of Birth (MM-DD-YYYY) 06/20/1978 Age 25 years

Sex (M/F) M On medication (Y/N) N

Diagnosis 1 (ICD code) Medication A
Diagnosis 2 (ICD code) Medication B
Diagnosis 3 (ICD code) Medication C

Test Version 4.2 TEST INFORMATION

Group Code ID Code Examiner Code

Date 02/26/2004 10:59AM Note

Comment

Brain Train 02/26/2004 10:59AM

Auditory Raw	Auditory Quotient	RESPONSE CONTROL Primary Scales	Visual Quotient	Visual Raw
96.0%	86	Prudence	101	96.9%
80.4%	97	Consistency	109	81.7%
83.0%	68	Stamina	93	97.1%
Hyperactive Events: 0			Fine Motor Reg. Quot: 110	

Auditory Raw	Auditory Quotient	ATTENTION Primary Scales	Visual Quotient	Visual Raw
100.0%	107	Vigilance	106	100.0%
78.4%	94	Focus	96	79.6%
598ms	97	Speed	97	434ms

Attribute		Raw	Q	<----+----+----o----+----+---->
Balance		72.6%	101	Vis Dom — No Bias — Aud Dom
Readiness	A	95.4%	105	A
	-			
	V	91.8%	98	V
				High — No Bias — Low

Symptomatic		Raw	Q	WNL Mild Mod Sev Ext
Comprehension	A	100.0%	103	A
	-			
	V	100.0%	103	V
Persistence	A	66.0%	73	A
	-			
	V	95.1%	97	V
Sensory/Motor	A	286ms	104	A
	-			
	V	272ms	88	V

Norms: IVA+Plus 2004.1 03-14-2001 for M age 25 - 29

Company	Cambridge Cognition
Location	Cambridge, United Kingdom
Website	www.cantabmobile.com
Cognitive Test Product	CANTABmobile
Test Features	
Testing Time	15 minutes or less
Testing Platform	Tablet - iPad
Can be Administered by Office Staff?	Yes, by qualified health care professionals.
Cognitive Domains Tested	Visual Episodic Memory, Psychomotor function
Test Primarily used for Detection of:	Mild Cognitive Impairment (MCI), Alzheimer's Disease, other dementia types
Test Validity and References	See Company End Notes Section for Test Validation References
Test Report Format	Standard scores Summary report – See sample next page.
Pricing Information	£100 per test ($150 US). Currently available only in the United Kingdom to licensed professionals. Contact company for other pricing.

CANTABmobile Test Report

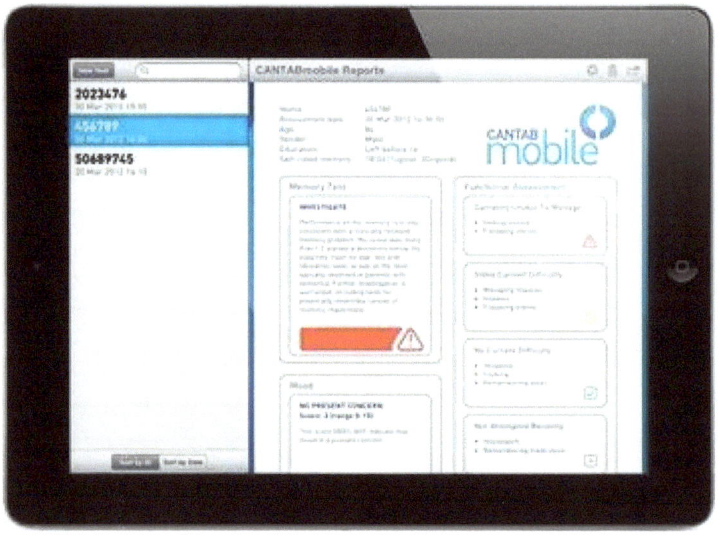

Investigate

Patient is below the norm expected of their age, gender and level of education indicative of a clinically relevant memory problem. If routine tests show no reversible cause for memory impairment, the patient should be referred on for further assessment.

Monitor

Performance on the memory test was at the lower end of the normative range. The patient may benefit from additional assessment or monitoring over time.

No present concern

Performance on the PAL memory test was in the normal range. There are no signs of memory impairment at this time. Reassess in the future if the patient notices a worsening of memory.

COMPANY	CNS VITAL SIGNS
LOCATION	Morrisville, North Carolina, USA
WEBSITE	www.cnsvs.com
COGNITIVE TEST PRODUCT	CNS Vital Signs
TEST FEATURES	
TESTING TIME	30 minutes
REQUIRED HARDWARE	Keyboard, monitor.
CAN BE ADMINISTERED BY OFFICE STAFF?	Yes, with training.
COGNITIVE DOMAINS TESTED	Memory, Processing Speed, Executive Function, Reaction Time, Complex Attention
TEST PRIMARILY USED FOR DETECTION OF:	Mild Cognitive Impairment (MCI), Alzheimer's Disease, other dementia types. Secondary use for neuropsychiatric disorders.
TEST VALIDITY AND REFERENCES	See Company End Notes Section for Test Validation References
TEST REPORT FORMAT	Standard scores Percentiles Raw scores for subtests See sample report next page.
PRICING INFORMATION	$25 per test when purchasing a block of ten tests.

CNS Vital Signs Clinical Report	Test Date: January 26, 2009 09:52:54
Subject ID: 02124	Administrator: TA Patient
Language: English (United States)	Age: 81
Total Test Time: 30:3 (min:secs)	Total time taken to complete all test in this report.

Above average domain scores indicate a standard score in that domain of greater than 109. Average is 90-109. Low Average is 80-89. Below Average is 70-79. Very Low is less than 70. Reaction times are in milliseconds. An * denotes that "lower is better", otherwise higher scores are better.

Patient Profile	Percentile Range			> 74	25 - 74	9 - 24	2 - 8	< 2
	Standard Score Range			> 109	90 - 109	80 - 89	70 - 79	< 70
Domain Scores	Subject Score	Standard Score	Percentile	Above	Average	Low Average	Low	Very Low
Composite Memory	92	108	70		X			
Verbal Memory	48	104	61		X			
Visual Memory	44	110	75	X				
Psychomotor Speed	120	102	55		X			
Reaction Time*	658	123	94	X				
Cognitive Flexibility	35	111	77	X				
Processing Speed	31	106	66		X			
Executive Functioning	35	111	77	X				

Verbal Memory Test (VBM)	Score	Standard	Percentile	
Correct Hits - Immediate	10	94	34	Memory test: Subjects have to remember 15 words and recognize them in a field of 15 distractors. The test is repeated at the end of the battery. "Correct Hits" refers to the number of target words recognized. Low scores indicate verbal memory impairment. Deficits in delayed recognition occur in patients with early dementia.
Correct Passes - Immediate	15	112	79	
Correct Hits - Delay	8	95	37	
Correct Passes - Delay	15	112	79	
Visual Memory Test (VSM)	**Score**	**Standard**	**Percentile**	
Correct Hits - Immediate	10	90	25	Memory test: Subjects have to remember 15 geometric figures and recognize them in a field of 15 distractors. The test is repeated at the end of the battery. "Correct Hits" refers to the number of target figures recognized. Low scores indicate visual memory impairment. Deficits in delayed recognition occur in patients with early dementia.
Correct Passes - Immediate	13	124	95	
Correct Hits - Delay	9	92	30	
Correct Passes - Delay	12	116	86	
Finger Tapping Test (FTT)	**Score**	**Standard**	**Percentile**	
Right Taps Average	44	100	50	Motor speed and fine motor control test: There are three rounds of tapping with each hand. Low scores indicate motor slowing. Most people are faster with their preferred hand but not always.
Left Taps Average	45	102	55	
Symbol Digit Coding (SDC)	**Score**	**Standard**	**Percentile**	
Correct Responses	31	103	58	Psychomotor speed and visual-motor coordination test: Errors may be due to impulsive responding, misperception or confusion. SDC is very sensitive to aging and also keyboarding skills. SDC is a two minute test.
Errors*	0	110	75	
Stroop Test (ST)	**Score**	**Standard**	**Percentile**	
Simple Reaction Time*	536	92	30	Processing speed, cognitive flexibility, and inhibition/disinhibition test: Prolonged reaction times indicate cognitive slowing/impairment. Errors may be due to impulsive responding, misperception or confusion. Reading disabilities may be apparent in this test. The ST generates simple and complex reaction times.
Complex Reaction Time Correct*	632	114	82	
Stroop Reaction Time Correct*	683	121	92	
Stroop Commission Errors*	0	110	75	
Shifting Attention Test (SAT)	**Score**	**Standard**	**Percentile**	
Correct Responses	40	107	68	Executive control and set shifting test: Subjects have to adjust their responses to randomly changing rules. The best scores are high correct responses, few errors and a short reaction time. Normal subjects may be slow but accurate, or fast but not so accurate. Attention deficit disabilities may be apparent.
Errors*	5	115	84	
Correct Reaction Time*	1183	110	75	

The CNS Vital Signs computerized neuropsychological assessment interpretation guide.

Additional information can be found on the CNS Vital Signs website: www.cnsvs.com

CNS Vital Signs VS7 clinical battery is a precise computerized assessment of neurocognitive status, which measures the speed and accuracy of five basic mental functions. These mental functions are indicators of the health and integrity of the brain's higher functions. The CNS Vital Signs report is used to evaluate and manage many neuro/psych conditions by:

Clinical Severity Grading (Single Administration) CPT Code: 96101/02/03/16 or 96118/19/20 CNS/Neurocognitive Tests The CNS Vital Signs computerized neuropsychological assessment can provide diagnostic clarification and grading of the clinical severity of impairment for patients with subclinical or obvious cognitive deficits. CNS Vital Signs is sensitive to the functional manifestations.

Monitoring and Grading Disease Progression (Serial Administration) CPT Code: 96101/02/03/16 or 96118/19/20 CNS/Neurocognitive Tests. CNS Vital Signs objectively documents and grades patient's neurocognitive status. Serial testing of impairment permits assessment of the progression of disease. This information guides the clinician's decision for the most appropriate treatment and/or referral.

Clarify or Confirm Diagnosis of Sub-clinical or Obvious Deficits(Single Administration) CPT Code: 96101/02/03/16 or 96118/19/20 CNS/Neurocognitive Tests. CNS Vital Signs can assist the clinician in clarifying the uncertainties in diagnosis. CNS Vital Signs also documents the status and degree of neurocognitive impairment before, during, and after treatment.

Medication ManagementCPT Code: 90862 Medication Management. With the advent of computerized neurocognitive tests such as CNS Vital Signs and medications designed to treat diseases characterized by cognitive dysfunction (e.g., Alzheimer's disease, epilepsy, attention deficit hyperactivity disorder, etc.), neurocognition has become a primary outcome measure for clinicians to use in the evaluation and management of their patients.

CNS Vital Signs Generates Profiles for Different Conditions Clinicians will recognize over time that each domain is sensitive to different clinical conditions. Clinicians will be able to compare age matched patients with MCI and dementia compared to norms as profiled on the report. The same utility exists for ADHD, brain injury, epilepsy and other neurological diseases. It is important to note that patients may experience global deficits or domain specific deficits across a variety of neurological disease states.

	Memory	Psychomotor Speed	Reaction Time	Complex Attention	Cognitive Flexibility
Mild Cognitive Impairment (MCI)	XX	X	X	XX	XX
Dementia	XX			XX	XX
Brain Injury		XX	X	X	XX
AD/HD			X	XX	XX
Depression		X	X	XX	XX
Executive Control Function			XX	XX	XX

XX	**Most Sensitive**	X	**Some Sensitive**		**Low Sensitive**

Evaluating Executive Control Function
Executive control functions refer to the capacity for autonomous behavior beyond the structure of external guidance. In clinical terms, this refers to initiative, motivation, spontaneity, planning, judgment, insight, goal-directed behavior, the ability to operate in favor of a remote or an abstract reward, the capacity for self-monitoring, and the flexibility required for self-correction. CNS Vital Signs has three tests that are sensitive to **executive control functions.**

Neurocognitive Domains Measured: The domain scores are computed from the seven neuropsychological tests. For a more fine-grained analysis examination the individual test scores may be needed.

Neurocognition Index (NCI) - An average of the five neurocognitive domains and a general assessment of the overall neurocognitive status of the patient. **Relevance:** Summary View.

Memory - Problems with the storage, manipulation and retrieval of information. The domain measures the ability to remember words and geometric figures. **Relevance:** Remembering, turning off the stove, recalling an appointment or rehabilitation information.

Psychomotor Speed - Problems with slowed information processing (i.e., perceiving, attending/responding to incoming information Motor speed, fine motor coordination, and visual-perceptual ability. **Relevance:** Medication effect.

Reaction Time - Problems with reacting to stimuli. Speed of reaction to complex directions (in milliseconds). **Relevance:** Driving a car, attending to conversation, tracking and responding to a set of simple instructions.

Complex Attention - Problems attending to multiple stimuli at the same time. Ability to maintain focus, track information over brief or lengthy periods of time, performs mental tasks quickly and accurately. **Relevance:** Self-regulation, learning, productivity.

Cognitive Flexibility - Problems shifting attention between two stimuli. Ability to adapt to rapidly changing directions and/or to manipulate the information. **Relevance:** Switching tasks, decision-making, impulse control, strategy formation.

Attention should be paid to both the nature and pattern of responses as well as to the quantity of errors committed. Patient's who score average or above average on all five domains are not likely to be impaired.

Patient's who score well below average in one domain or below average in two domain areas, might well be impaired and should be evaluated further. The first step, in evaluating such a patient is to repeat the test under more favorable circumstances.

If the scores are equally low the second time, a targeted work-up is necessary. **NORMAL AGING** affects performance on all of these tests; but the range of normal scores are based on data from normal controls who are the same age as the patient being tested. **EDUCATION and SPECIAL SKILLS** may also affect test performance; therefore, concern should be taken for patient's that are very intelligent or well educated yet their scores are below average. Patient's who are less intelligent, may score below average or well below average. These results, however, may be less meaningful. They may simply be a function of the patient's inherent weakness. Like any laboratory test, an abnormal result should be the occasion of a differential diagnosis, and further inquiry.

To Order Test Assessments GO TO: www.cnsvs.com, EMAIL: support@cnsvs.com, or PHONE the SUPPORT Line: 888.750.6941; OUTSIDE the USA 202.449.8492

Medical Outcomes Survey (MOS) SF-36 (page 1 of 2)

Subject Reference/ID: 02124	Test Date: January 26, 2009 09:52:54
Age: 81	Administrator: TA Patient
Total Test Time: 30:3 (min:secs) for all tests in this report	Language: English (United States)
This scale was administered using CNS Vital Signs	

Domain	Score	Standard	Percentile
Physical Functioning	35	81	10
Role Functioning/Physical	50	99	47
Role Functioning/Emotional	100	113	81
Energy/Fatigue	30	85	16
Emotional Wellbeing	76	104	61
Social Functioning	100	113	81
Pain	68	98	45
General Health	20	74	4
Health Change	25	78	7

As part of the Medical Outcomes Survey (MOS) - a multi-year, multi-site study to explain variations in patient outcomes - RAND (www.rand.org) developed the 36-Item Medical Outcomes Survey (SF-36). SF-36 is a set of generic, coherent, and easily administered quality-of-life measures. These measures rely upon patient self-reporting and are now widely utilized by managed care organizations and by Medicare for routine monitoring and assessment of care outcomes in adult patients.

Medical Outcomes Short Form Health Survey (SF-36) Questions

1	In general, would you say your health is:	Fair
2	Compared to one year ago, how would you rate your health in general now?	Somewhat worse now than one year ago

The following items are about activities you might do during a typical day. Does your health now limit you in these activities? If so, how much?

3	Vigorous activities, such as running lifting heavy objects, participating in strenuous sports	Yes, limited a lot
4	Moderate activities, such as moving a table, pushing a vacuum cleaner, bowling or playing golf	Yes, limited a lot
5	Lifting or carrying groceries	No, not limited at all
6	Climbing several flights of stairs	Yes, limited a lot
7	Climbing one flight of stairs	Yes, limited a lot
8	Bending, kneeling, or stooping	Yes, limited a lot
9	Walking more than a mile	Yes, limited a lot
10	Walking several blocks	Yes, limited a little
11	Walking one block	No, not limited at all
12	Bathing or dressing yourself	No, not limited at all

During the past 4 weeks, have you had any of the following problems with your work or other regular daily activities as a result of your physical health?

13	Cut down on the amount of time you spent on work or other actvities	No
14	Accomplished less than you would like	Yes
15	Were limited in the kind of work or other activities	No
16	Had difficulty performing the work or other activities (for example, it took extra effort)	Yes

During the past 4 weeks, have you had any of the following problems with your work or other regular daily activities as a result of any emotional problems (such as feeling depressed or anxious)?

17	Cut down on the amount of time you spent on work or other actvities	No
18	Accomplished less than you would like	No
19	Didn't do work or other activities as carefully as usual	No

During the past 4 weeks, to what extent has your physical health or emotional problems interfered with ...

20	your normal social activities with family, friends, neighbors, or groups?	Not at all

During the past 4 weeks ...

21	How much bodily pain have you had?	Mild
22	How much did pain interfere with your normal work (including both work outside the home and housework)?	Slightly

Medical Outcomes Survey (MOS) SF-36 (page 2 of 2)	
Subject Reference/ID: 02124	Test Date: January 26, 2009 09:52:54
Age: 81	Administrator: TA Patient
Total Test Time: 30:3 (min:secs) for all tests in this report	Language: English (United States)
This scale was administered using CNS Vital Signs	

These questions are about how you feel and how things have been with you during the past 4 weeks. For each question, please give the one answer that comes closest to the way you have been feeling. How much of the time during the past 4 weeks ...

23	Did you feel full of pep?	Some of the time
24	Have you been a very nervous person?	A little of the time
25	Have you felt so down in the dumps that nothing could cheer you up?	A little of the time
26	Have you felt calm and peaceful?	A good bit of the time
27	Did you have a lot of energy?	None of the time
28	Have you felt downhearted and blue?	Some of the time
29	Did you feel worn out?	A good bit of the time
30	Have you been a happy person?	All of the time
31	Did you feel tired?	A good bit of the time

During the past 4 weeks, how much of the time has your physical health or emotional problems interfered with ...

32	your social actvities (like visiting with friends, relatives, etc.)?	None of the time

How TRUE or FALSE is the following statement for you.

33	I seem to get sick a little easier than other people	Mostly false
34	I am as healthy as anybody I know	Definitely false
35	I expect my health to get worse	Definitely true
36	My health is excellent	Definitely false

COMPANY	COGSTATE
LOCATION	Melbourne, Australia
WEBSITE	www.cognigram.com
COGNITIVE TEST PRODUCT	COGNIGRAM

TEST FEATURES

TESTING TIME	30 minutes or less
TESTING PLATFORM	PC, keyboard, monitor. Internet connection required for test reporting.
CAN BE ADMINISTERED BY OFFICE STAFF?	Yes, by qualified health care professionals. Test is administered only in specialized testing centers.
COGNITIVE DOMAINS TESTED	Working Memory, Attention, Visual Memory, Psychomotor function
TEST PRIMARILY USED FOR DETECTION OF:	Mild Cognitive Impairment (MCI), Alzheimer's Disease, other dementia types
TEST VALIDITY AND REFERENCES	See Company End Notes Section for Test Validation References
TEST REPORT FORMAT	Standard scores Temporal (longitudinal) charts
PRICING INFORMATION	$125 CAD. Currently available only in Canada. Contact company for other availability and pricing.

COMPANY	HEADMINDER, INC.
LOCATION	New York City, New York, USA
WEBSITE	www.headminder.com
COGNITIVE TEST PRODUCT	Cognitive Stability Index (CST)
TEST FEATURES	
TESTING TIME	15 minutes
REQUIRED HARDWARE	Internet connection required, keyboard.
CAN BE ADMINISTERED BY OFFICE STAFF?	Yes, with training.
COGNITIVE DOMAINS TESTED	Memory, Learning, Attention, Processing Speed
TEST PRIMARILY USED FOR DETECTION OF:	Mild Cognitive Impairment (MCI), Alzheimer's Disease, other dementia types
TEST VALIDITY AND REFERENCES	See Company End Notes Section for Test Validation References
TEST REPORT FORMAT	Impairment Index Summary Standard Scores for subtests See sample report next page
PRICING INFORMATION	Contact Company

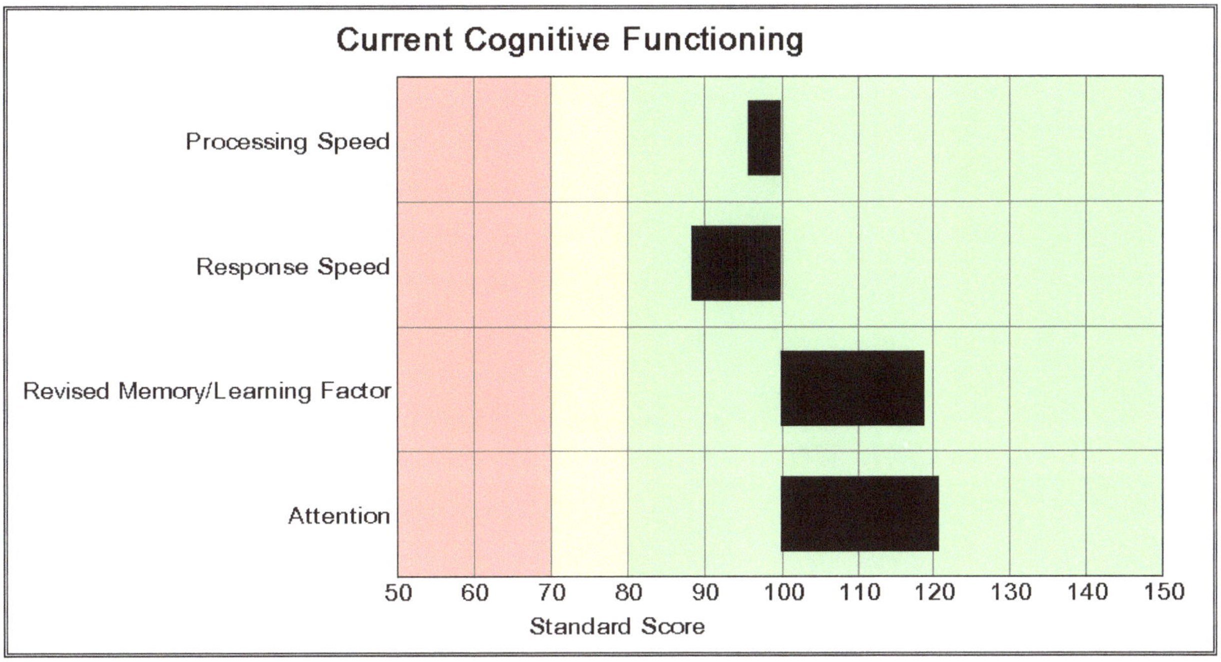

Standard Score Explanation:
The horizontal bars depict how much lower or higher than average a person scored by means of a standard score. A standard score is derived from an individual's raw score after adjusting for age and other demographic variables and allows comparison to a normative group. The average standard score is 100 and the standard deviation is 15. This means that 68% of all normal [uninjured] test takers will obtain a score between 85 and 115 (+/- 1 st dev) and 96% will obtain a score between 70 and 130 (+/- 2 st dev).

Subtest Scores

Factor / Subtest	Result	Range	Standard Score	Percentile
Processing Speed				
Animal Decoding - Number Correct	✓	Average	96	39th
Symbol Scanning - Average Response Time	✓	Below Average	87	19th
Response Speed				
Response Direction 1 - Average Response Time	✓	Below Average	86	18th
Response Direction 1 - Errors	✓	Average		> 8th
Response Direction 2 - Average Response Time	✓	Below Average	83	13th
Response Direction 2 - Errors	✓	Average		> 8th
Incidental Learning 1 - Average Response Time	✓	Average	102	54th
Incidental Learning 1 - Errors	✓	Average		> 8th
Incidental Learning 2 - Average Response Time	✓	Below Average	86	18th
Incidental Learning 2 - Errors	✓	Average		> 8th
Revised Memory/Learning Factor				

Incidental Learning 2 - Number Correct	✓	Above Average	111	76th
Memory Cabinet 1 - Number Correct	✓	Above Average	113	81st
Memory Cabinet 2 - Number Correct	✓	Above Average	111	76th
Attention				
Number Recall - Number Correct	✓	Above Average	126	96th
Number Sequencing - Number Correct	✓	Above Average	111	76th

✓ indicates a score in the acceptable range.

! or ⓔ indicates a score in the borderline range.

! or ⓔ indicates a score in the impaired range.

Note: Some individuals may have impaired subtest scores, but factor scores within normal limits. Clinical judgment is required to determine the relevance of isolated impaired range test scores.
See the *CSI Professional Manual* for a discussion.

Company	ImPACT Applications, Inc.
Location	Pittsburgh, Pennsylvania USA
Website	www.impacttest.com
Cognitive Test Product	ImPACT Concussion Assessment
Test Features	
Testing Time	20 minutes
Testing Platform	PC, Monitor, Keyboard. Internet connection required.
Can be Administered by Office Staff?	Yes, after receiving training on ImPACT test administration.
Cognitive Domains Tested	Attention, Working Memory, Response Inhibition, Reaction Time, Processing Speed
Test Primarily used for Detection of:	Concussion symptoms
Test Validity and References	See Company End Notes Section for Test Validation References
Test Report Format	Summary and detail scores. See sample report next page.
Pricing Information	$10 per baseline assessment test. $20 per post-injury assessment test.

Mark

Organization:	**Sample Hockey Team**		
Subject ID#:	**111-22-3333**		
Date of birth:	**01/01/86**	Age:	**19**
Gender:	**Male**	Height:	**73** inches
Handedness:	**Right**	Weight:	**190** lbs
Native country / region:	**Canada**	Second language:	**(None)**
Native language:	**English**	Years speaking:	**0**
Years of education completed excluding kindergarten:	**12**	Received speech therapy:	**No**
Diagnosed learning disability:	**No**	Problems with ADD/Hyperactivity:	**No**
Attended special education classes:	**No**	Repeated one or more years of school:	**No**
Current sport:	**Hockey**	Current level of participation:	**OHL**
Primary position/event/class:	**LW/C**	Years experience at this level:	**2**

Number of times diagnosed with a concussion (excluding current injury):	**1**
Concussions that resulted in loss of conciousness:	**0**
Concussions that resulted in confusion:	**0**
Concussions that resulted in difficulty remembering events that occured immediately after injury:	**0**
Concussions that resulted in difficulty remembering events that occured	**0**
Total games missed as a result of all concussions combined:	**0**

Concussion history: **10/07/2004**

Treatment for headaches by physician:	**No**	Treatment for psychiatric condition (depression, anxiety):	**No**
Treatment for epilepsy / seizures:	**No**	Treatment for migraine headaches by physician:	**No**
History of brain surgery:	**No**	Treatment for substance/alcohol abuse:	**No**
History of meningitis:	**No**		

ImPACT© Clinical Report

Mark

Exam Type	Baseline	Post-concussion	Post-concussion	Post-concussion	Post-concussion	Post-concussion
Date Tested	09/21/2004	10/08/2004	10/12/2004	10/15/2004	10/19/2004	10/27/2004
Last Concussion		10/07/2004	10/07/2004	10/07/2004	10/07/2004	10/07/2004
Exam Language	English	English	English	English	English	English
Test Version	2.2.729	2.2.729	2.2.729	2.2.729	2.2.729	2.2.729

Composite Scores *												
Memory composite (verbal)	93	75%	**66**	1%	**57**	<1%	**63**	<1%	87	55%	88	55%
Memory composite (visual)†	70	23%	**41**	<1%	**49**	1%	**47**	<1%	**55**	3%	66	12%
Visual motor speed composite	45.88	85%	46.38	86%	**40.13**	65%	**38.93**	57%	45.85	85%	41.90	72%
Reaction time composite	0.54	46%	0.60	22%	**0.66**	6%	0.54	46%	**0.62**	15%	0.54	46%
Impulse control composite	8		14		10		16		10		11	
Total Symptom Score	0		**14**		3		1		0		0	

* Scores in **bold** type indicate scores that exceed the Reliable Change Index score (RCI) when compared to the baseline score. However, scores that do not exceed the RCI index may still be clinically significant. Percentile scores, if available, are listed in small type. Please consult your ImPACT User Manual for more details.

† Clinical composite score is available only for exams taken in ImPACT version 2.0 or later.

Concussion Details	
Date of concussion	10/07/2004
Loss of consciousness	None
Retrograde amnesia	None
Anterograde amnesia	None
Confusion / disorientation	None
Returned to play	Did not return
Taken to hospital	
CT/MRI scan of head	None
Point of impact	
Mouthguard type	Vacuum form
Mouthguard condition	Good
Mouthguard manufacturer	
Helmet manufacturer	
Helmet model	
Helmet size	
Symptoms	headache, dizziness or balance problems
Description of injury and additional information	Was hit from behind into the boards by an opposing player. He went in almost head first.

The information provided by this report should be viewed as only one source of information regarding the athlete's level o functioning. Diagnostic or return to play decisions should not be based solely on the data generated by ImPACT but should be basec on an evaluation made by qualified medical personnel in accordance with usual and standard medical practice. If an individual is suspected of suffering a mild traumatic brain injury or concussion, this individual should be evaluated by medical personnel anc should be followed carefully for the emergence of symptoms.

Consultation is recommended to help facilitate proper interpretation of the information provided by this report. For initial post-injur consultation you are urged to contact Dr. Mark Lovell or Dr. Micky Collins at ImPACT Applications. To reinforce proper interpretatior of the test data, there will be no charge for the intial post-injury consultation.

Dr. Mark Lovell can be reached at:
412-432-3670 (Office)
412-432-3681 (Secretary)
lovellmr@upmc.edu

Dr. Micky Collins can be reached at:
412-432-3668 (Office)
412-958-6714 (Pager)
collinsmw@upmc.edu

Exam Type	Baseline	Post-concussion	Post-concussion	Post-concussion	Post-concussion	Post-concussion
Date Tested	09/21/2004	10/08/2004	10/12/2004	10/15/2004	10/19/2004	10/27/2004
Last Concussion		10/07/2004	10/07/2004	10/07/2004	10/07/2004	10/07/2004

Word Memory	*WG = 1*	*WG = 2*	*WG = 3*	*WG = 4*	*WG = 5*	*WG = 4*
Hits (immediate)	12	11	9	11	11	12
Correct distractors (immed.)	12	11	10	12	12	12
Learning percent correct	100%	92%	79%	96%	96%	100%
Hits (delay)	11	9	8	4	5	10
Correct distractors (delay)	8	6	5	10	7	7
Delayed memory pct. correct	79%	63%	54%	58%	50%	71%
Total percent correct	90%	77%	67%	77%	73%	85%

Design Memory						
Hits (immediate)	8	7	9	5	8	11
Correct distractors (immed.)	9	9	5	8	9	10
Learning percent correct	71%	67%	58%	54%	71%	88%
Hits (delay)	9	9	8	7	9	8
Correct distractors (delay)	9	2	5	5	7	6
Delayed memory pct. correct	75%	46%	54%	50%	67%	58%
Total percent correct	73%	56%	56%	52%	69%	73%

X's and O's						
Total correct (memory)	8	3	5	5	5	7
Total correct (interference)	115	107	93	105	110	112
Avg. correct RT (interference)	0.45	0.45	0.64	0.47	0.48	0.46
Total incorrect (interference)	7	14	8	14	8	10
Avg. incorrect RT (interfer.)	0.37	0.37	0.50	0.40	0.44	0.37

Symbol Match						
Total correct (visible)	27	27	27	27	27	26
Avg. correct RT (visible)	1.19	1.42	1.39	1.19	1.29	1.22
Total correct (hidden)	8	5	4	6	8	7
Avg. correct RT (hidden)	1.06	1.38	1.18	1.52	1.38	1.08

Color Match						
Total correct	9	9	8	9	9	9
Avg. correct RT	0.78	0.87	0.89	0.76	0.94	0.75
Total commissions	1	0	2	2	2	1
Avg. commissions RT	0.57	0.00	1.68	0.54	0.49	0.99

Three Letters						
Total sequence correct	5	2	2	1	5	5
Total letters correct	15	10	9	7	15	15
Pct. of total letters correct	100%	67%	60%	47%	100%	100%
Avg. time to first click	1.95	2.42	1.89	1.70	1.21	1.91
Avg. counted	21.2	22.0	20.0	19.2	21.2	21.2
Avg. counted correctly	21.0	22.0	19.0	17.2	21.4	18.6

Exam Type	Baseline	Post-concussion	Post-concussion	Post-concussion	Post-concussion	Post-concussion
Date Tested	09/21/2004	10/08/2004	10/12/2004	10/15/2004	10/19/2004	10/27/2004
Last Concussion		10/07/2004	10/07/2004	10/07/2004	10/07/2004	10/07/2004
Headache	0	2	1	0	0	0
Nausea	0	0	0	0	0	0
Vomiting	0	0	0	0	0	0
Balance Problems	0	0	0	0	0	0
Dizziness	0	1	0	0	0	0
Fatigue	0	2	0	0	0	0
Trouble falling asleep	0	2	0	0	0	0
Sleeping more than usual	0	0	0	0	0	0
Sleeping less than usual	0	2	0	0	0	0
Drowsiness	0	0	0	0	0	0
Sensitivity to light	0	0	0	0	0	0
Sensitivity to noise	0	1	0	0	0	0
Irritability	0	2	0	0	0	0
Sadness	0	0	0	0	0	0
Nervousness	0	0	0	0	0	0
Feeling more emotional	0	0	0	0	0	0
Numbness or tingling	0	0	0	0	0	0
Feeling slowed down	0	1	0	0	0	0
Feeling mentally foggy	0	1	1	0	0	0
Difficulty concentrating	0	0	1	1	0	0
Difficulty remembering	0	0	0	0	0	0
Visual problems	0	0	0	0	0	0
Total Symptom Score	**0**	**14**	**3**	**1**	**0**	**0**

The information provided by this report should be viewed as only one source of information regarding the athlete's level of functioning. Diagnostic or return to play decisions should not be based solely on the data generated by ImPACT but should be based on an evaluation made by qualified medical personnel in accordance with usual and standard medical practice. If an individual is suspected of suffering a mild traumatic brain injury or concussion, this individual should be evaluated by medical personnel and should be followed carefully for the emergence of symptoms.

Consultation is recommended to help facilitate proper interpretation of the information provided by this report. For initial post-injury consultation you are urged to contact Dr. Mark Lovell or Dr. Micky Collins at ImPACT Applications. To reinforce proper interpretation of the test data, there will be no charge for the intial post-injury consultation.

Dr. Mark Lovell can be reached at:
412-432-3670 (Office)
412-432-3681 (Secretary)
lovellmr@upmc.edu

Dr. Micky Collins can be reached at:
412-432-3668 (Office)
412-958-6714 (Pager)
collinsmw@upmc.edu

Baseline	Hours slept last night	8.0
09/21/2004	Medication	
	Subject comments	ENVIRONMENT: constant noise in background
	Supervisor comments	

Post-concussion	Hours slept last night	6.0
10/08/2004	Medication	
	Subject comments	ENVIRONMENT: background noise
	Supervisor comments	

Post-concussion	Hours slept last night	8.0
10/12/2004	Medication	
	Subject comments	ENVIRONMENT: background noise
	Supervisor comments	

Post-concussion	Hours slept last night	8.0
10/15/2004	Medication	
	Subject comments	
	Supervisor comments	

Post-concussion	Hours slept last night	9.0
10/19/2004	Medication	
	Subject comments	ENVIRONMENT: constant interuptions
	Supervisor comments	

Post-concussion	Hours slept last night	9.0
10/27/2004	Medication	
	Subject comments	
	Supervisor comments	

Dr. Mark Lovell can be reached at:
412-432-3670 (Office)
412-432-3681 (Secretary)
lovellmr@upmc.edu

Dr. Micky Collins can be reached at:
412-432-3668 (Office)
412-958-6714 (Pager)
collinsmw@upmc.edu

Memory Composite (Verbal)

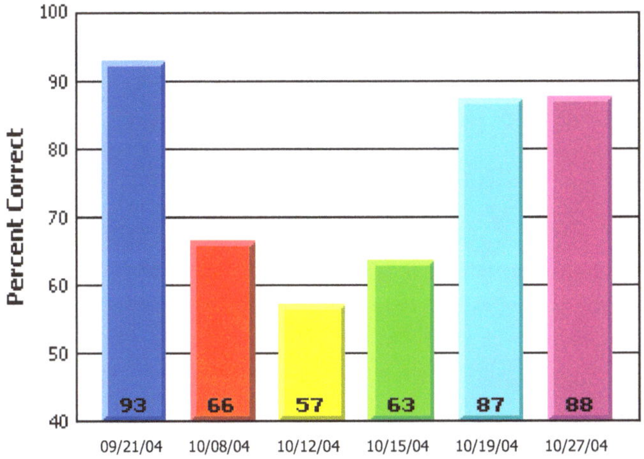

Memory Composite (Visual)

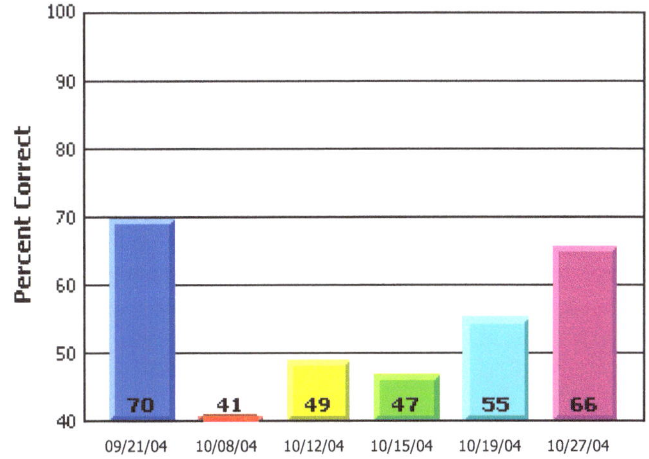

Visual Motor Speed Composite

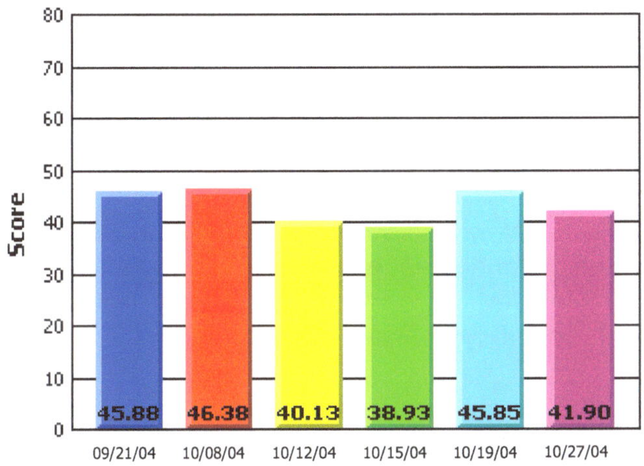

Reaction Time Composite

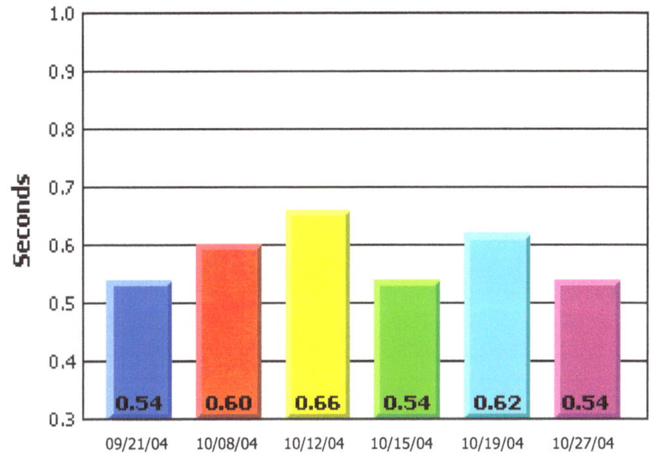

Impulse Control Composite

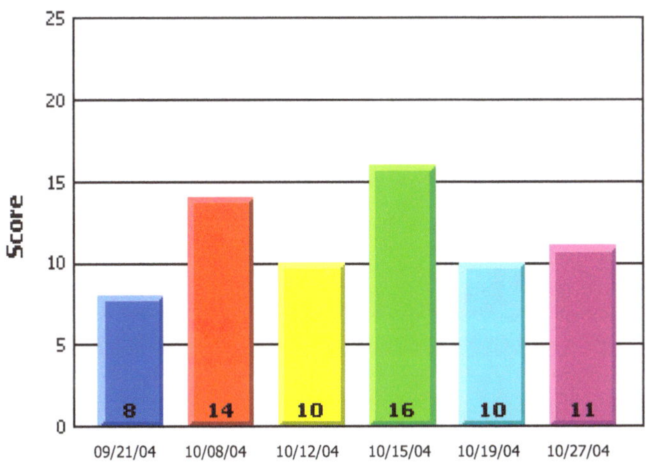

Symptom Score

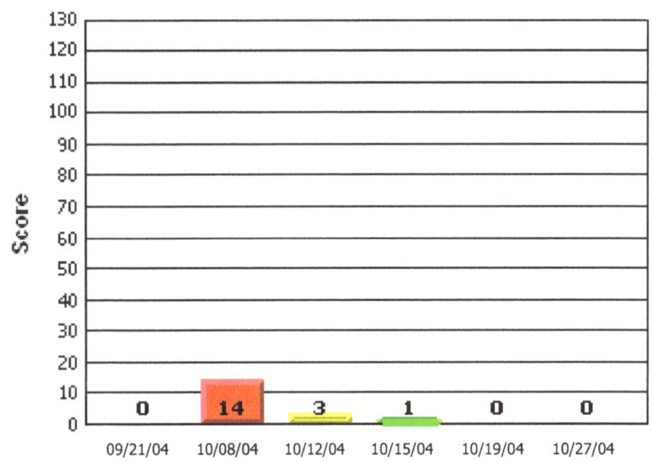

COMPANY	MEDICAL CARE CORP.
LOCATION	Newport Beach, California, USA
WEBSITE	www.mccare.com
COGNITIVE TEST PRODUCT	MCI Screen
TEST FEATURES	
TESTING TIME	8-12 minutes
REQUIRED HARDWARE	**For test scoring only**: internet connection required. Any method of data entry will work (IPAD, keyboard, touch screen, mouse)
CAN BE ADMINISTERED BY OFFICE STAFF?	Yes. One online practice session required. Reliability compared to neuropsychologist = 0.83 (Trenkle et al. 2007).
COGNITIVE DOMAINS TESTED	Episodic Memory, Working Memory, Judgement, Serial Position Effects, Attention, Comprehension, Metamemory, Delayed Recognition Memory, Rehearsed and Unrehearsed Delayed Free Recall.
TEST PRIMARILY USED FOR DETECTION OF:	Mild Cognitive Impairment (MCI), Alzheimer's Disease, other dementia types
TEST VALIDITY AND REFERENCES	Test Sensitivity for MCI = 95%, Test Specificity for Normal Aging = 88% Test Sensitivity for Mild Dementia = 96%, Specificity for Normal Aging = 99%
TEST REPORT FORMAT	Summary Percentile Rank Standard Scores Raw Scores for subtests See sample report next page
PRICING INFORMATION	$29 per test

MCI Screen Report

Monday, May 21, 2012 11:25 AM

Subject	Patient Name		
DOB	1/1/45	**Gender**	Male
Age	67	**Education (yrs)**	16

Overall Impression: Below Normal

Memory Performance Index: 43

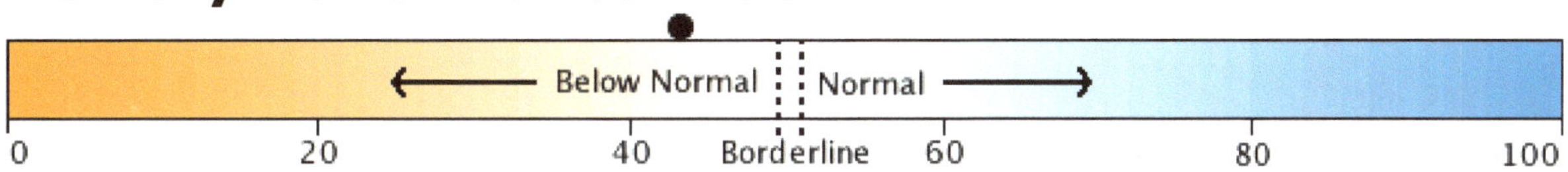

For the scores in the Below Normal range (0 ≤ MPI ≤ 49.8), smaller values indicate worse performance when compared to an individual's peers after accounting for effects of age, gender and education. For example, a score of 10 indicates worse cognitive performance than a score of 15.

Component		Status	Score/Max Score	Standardized Score [?]	Interpretation [?]
Memory Performance Index	[?]	Calculated	43/100	N/A	Below Normal
Recall Pattern	[?]	Analyzed	N/A	N/A	Below Normal
Immediate Recall Total	[?]	Understands	9/30	-3.4	Below Normal
Delayed Recall Estimate	[?]	Complete	7.5/10	N/A	Moderate Overestimate
Delayed Free Recall	[?]	Complete	3/10	-2.4	Below Normal
Delayed Cued Recall-Yes	[?]	Understands	5/10	-9.6	Below Normal
Delayed Cued Recall-No	[?]	Understands	9/10	-1.6	Below Normal
Animal Recall	[?]	Complete	4/9	N/A	N/A

Overall Finding
The patient's performance on the MCI Screen falls below the normal range compared to a demographically similar peer group.

Objective Findings
3 Cognitive Problems: Judgment, Working and Short-Term Memory Encoding

The patient had difficulty recalling a list of 10 words immediately (impaired attention or working memory), and after a delay of several minutes both with and without a 20 word list to choose from (impaired encoding into and retrieval from short term memory). The patient also had difficulty estimating his/her short term memory ability (impaired judgment or insight).

The MCI Screen is intended to provide a general assessment of memory function. It is not intended to diagnose or treat medical conditions or diseases that may contribute to memory function. This

assessment is limited to use by licensed medical professionals and is not a subsitute for professional medical advise. If seeking medical assistance, please consult with a healthcare professional.

Company	MedInteract
Location	Knoxville, Tennessee, USA
Website	www.medinteract.com
Cognitive Test Product	COGselftest
Test Features	
Testing Time	10 minutes
Required Hardware	Internet connection required, keyboard, mouse – or-touchscreen
Can be Administered by Office Staff?	Yes, with training.
Cognitive Domains Tested	Memory, Attention, Visual-Spatial Construction, Verbal Fluency, Processing Speed
Test Primarily used for Detection of:	Mild Cognitive Impairment (MCI), Alzheimer's Disease, other dementia types
Test Validity and References	See Company End Notes Section for Test Validation References.
Test Report Format	Raw Scores with norm comparison See sample report next page
Pricing Information	$25 per test. Volume discounts available.

Results of your COGselftest

Thank you for taking the COGSelftest, a web-based cognitive screening test. Studies have shown this online test to be 96% accurate in the screening for cognitive impairment in six areas: verbal fluency, attention, orientation, executive function, visual spatial, and memory.

Your test results have been saved under your account. To access these results in the future, simply log in and access your account.

Test results for May 6th, 2013, 3:59pm. Your results indicate warning markers in Orientation, Attention, Verbal Fluency, Memory, and Visual Spatial and Executive Functions. Since you missed questions in multiple cognitive domains, it is recommended that you print your results and take them to your physician for further evaluation. Your physician will be able to access our site for further details and information about your test (with your permission). Again, this is an early warning screening test, not a diagnosis. Only your physician can make a diagnosis. But we can help educate you and family members about scientifically proven ways to delay symptoms of cognitive impairment. That's why we are here.

Recent studies have shown there are many ways to keep our brains stimulated and our mental function optimal. Once you have reviewed your results below, click on each domain to learn more and print out the exercises to keep your mental function and peak performance. And be sure to sign up for our newsletter to stay up to date on the latest news and research on Alzheimer's Disease.

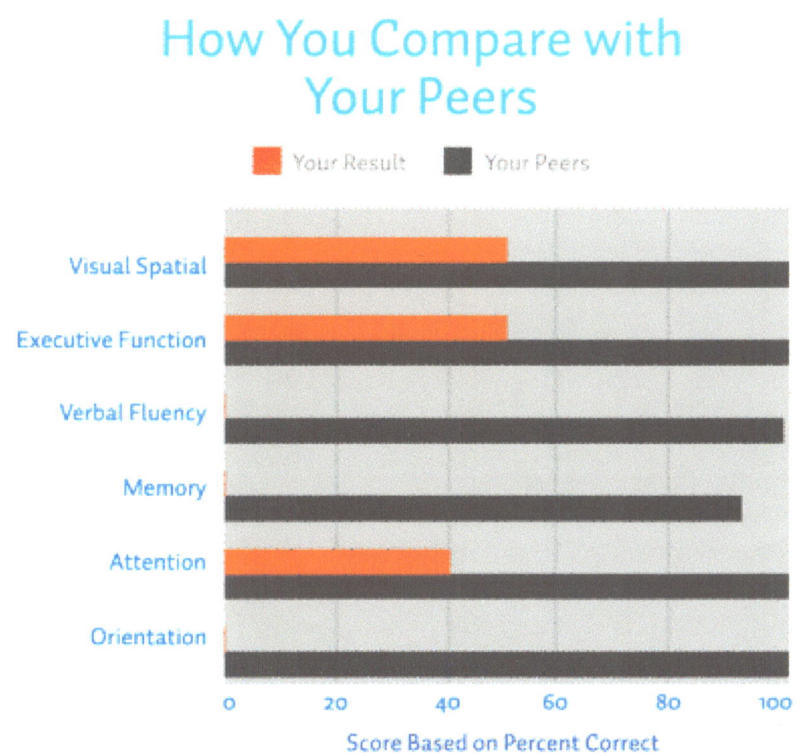

Results by Cognitive Domain

01.	Visuo-Spatial	MILD IMPAIRMENT
02.	Executive Functions	MILD IMPAIRMENT
03.	Verbal Fluency	NEEDS IMPROVEMENT
04.	Memory	NEEDS IMPROVEMENT
05.	Attention	MILD IMPAIRMENT
06.	Orientation	NEEDS IMPROVEMENT
07.	Processing Speed	EXCELLENT

Decode Your Results

Excellent: No problems flagged. Retake the test in six months.

Needs Improvement: Repeat test in three to six months. Consult Physician.

Below Average: Repeat test in three months. See Physician soon.

Please understand that no single test can make a definitive diagnosis of Alzheimer's Disease or other type of dementia. It is very important that you consult your physician for further evaluation. In order to receive a complete diagnosis, you must see your physician for a comprehensive exam, which will include a physical examination, blood tests, a thorough medical history, and more.

CST MEAN SCORE:

25

STANDARD DEVIATION 1.20, MINIMUM 22, MAXIMUM 27

(2) Early Alzheimer's Disease (EAD):

Early AD is characterized by neurocognitive deficits in two or more cognitive domains. Early AD typically involves impairment in several cognitive domains, with memory being the most likely to show significant deficits. Repeating oneself and asking the same question over again is frequently one of the earliest signs of Alzheimer's disease.

Difficulty in traveling to a new location and decreased organizational capacity are early symptoms, as well as difficulty in paying bills, writing checks and balancing the checkbook. Medications are very important at this stage of impairment, and further monitoring is vital to the overall care and quality of life for the patient.

Another area of concern is an individual's reaction to a negative report of memory problems or other cognitive symptoms. In our database, however, 48% of the Early AD group manifests symptoms of anosognosia (unawareness) of memory or other cognitive deficits. In Early AD, activities of daily living may or may not be compromised, and frequently objective confirmation of the clinical history may be necessary. In this stage, the clinical examination and neuroimaging data are often critical in confirming the diagnosis.

NEUROCOGNITIVE DOMAIN MEAN RAW SCORES FOR ALL EAD GROUPS IN CST DATABASE:

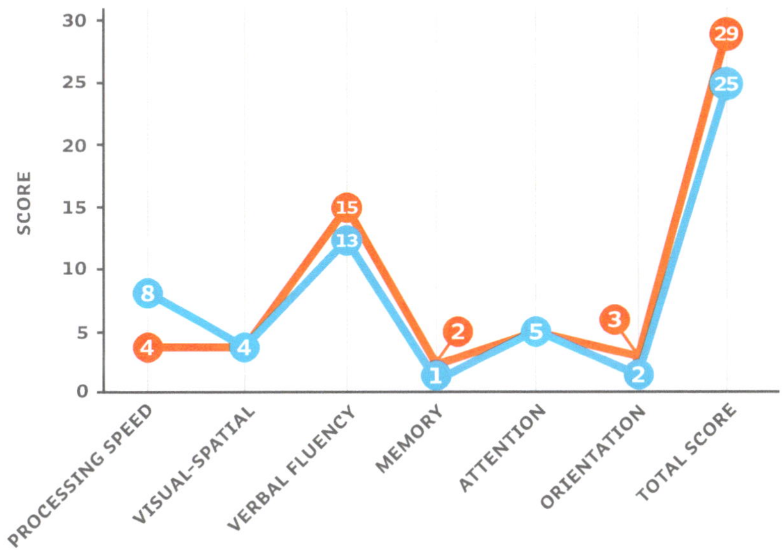

SUMMARY: NOTICEABLE DIFFERENCES BETWEEN THE CONTROL GROUP AND PATIENTS WITH EARLY ALZHEIMER'S DISEASE ARE FOUND IN THEIR PROCESSING SPEEDS, VERBAL FLUENCY, MEMORY AND ORIENTATION.

LEGEND:

EARLY ALZHEIMER'S DISEASE

CONTROL GROUP

Company	NeuroTrax
Location	Houston, Texas, USA
Website	www.neurotrax.com
Cognitive Test Product	MindStreams
Test Features	
Testing Time	15-30 minutes, depending on test battery
Required Hardware	Standard PC running XP/Vista/Windows 7, keyboard, USB mouse. Internet connection for report creation.
Can be Administered by Office Staff?	Yes, with training.
Cognitive Domains Tested	Memory (verbal & non-verbal), Executive Function, Attention, Information Processing Speed, Visual Spatial Processing, Verbal Function, Motor Skills
Test Primarily Used for Detection of:	Mild Cognitive Impairment (MCI), Alzheimer's Disease, other dementia types. Secondary use for neuropsychiatric disorders.
Test Validity and References	In a recent study, MindStreams correctly classified 89% of MCI individuals as converters or non-converters to early AD. See End Notes Section for further detail.
Test Report Format	Standard scores Raw scores See sample report next page.
Pricing Information	Costs range between $30-$50, depending on test battery. Volume discounts apply.

NeuroTrax® Mindstreams® Assessment Report

Advanced Cognitive Health Assessment www.mindstreamshealth.com

Patient Name: John Doe, ID 999999999
Date Of Birth: January 1, 1938
Referring Physician: Dr. Marcus Welby
Reason for Referral: Routine Cognitive Health Check-Up

Recent Dates of Testing

1. August 7, 2006, 11:13 AM
2. August 16, 2007, 9:42 AM
3. August 23, 2008, 10:03 AM
4. August 30, 2009, 9:57 AM

Testing Battery: Global Assessment Battery
Tests Included: Go-NoGo, Verbal Memory, Problem Solving, Stroop Interference, Non-Verbal Memory, Finger Tapping, Catch Game, Staged Info Proc, Visual Spatial Processing, Verbal Function

Cognitive Profile

Aug-30-09

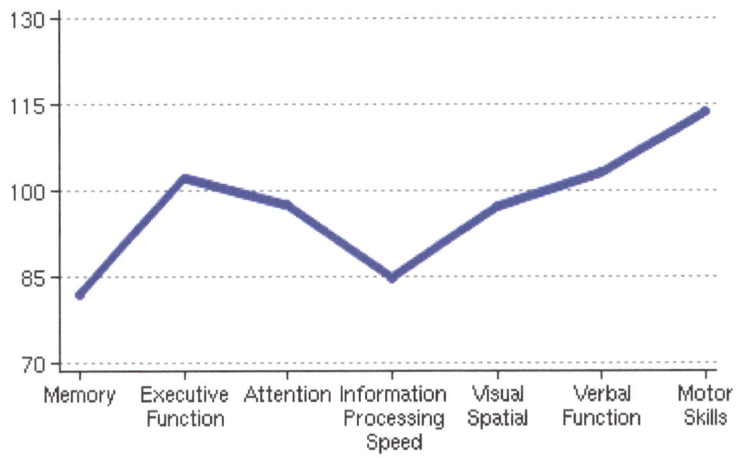

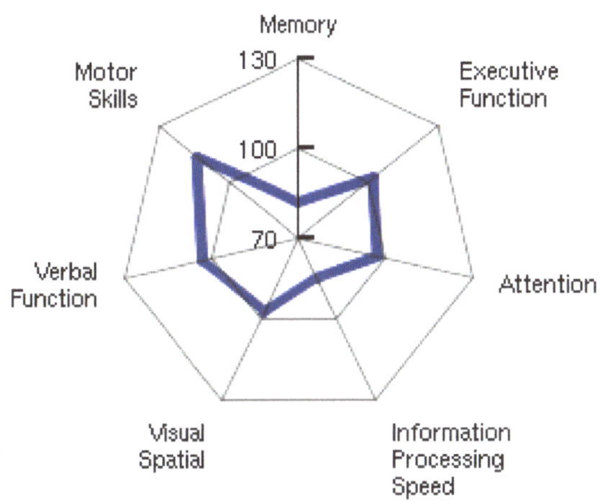

Global Cognitive Score: 97.2

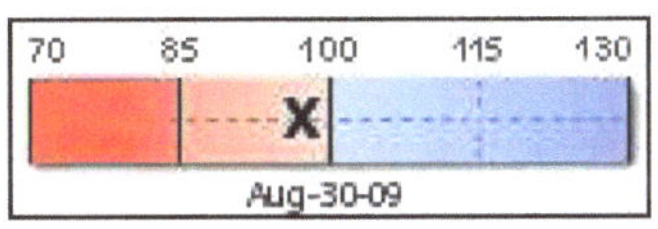

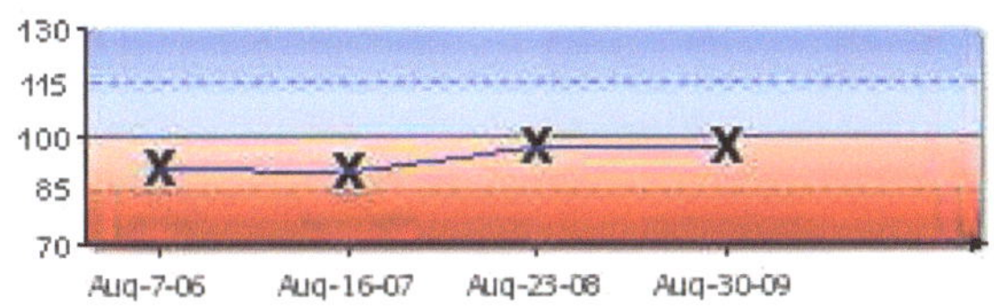

Summary

Relative to a population matched for age and education, performance on the present testing session was indicative of:

- Cognitive performance below 1 standard deviation from the average in the following cognitive domain(s): *Memory*, *Information Processing Speed*.
- Below average cognitive performance in the following cognitive domain(s): *Attention*, *Visual Spatial*.
- Above average cognitive performance in the following cognitive domain(s): *Executive Function*, *Verbal Function*, *Motor Skills*.
- **Global Cognitive Function** - Below average cognitive performance.

See "Interpretation of Performance Graphs" below.

Memory: 82

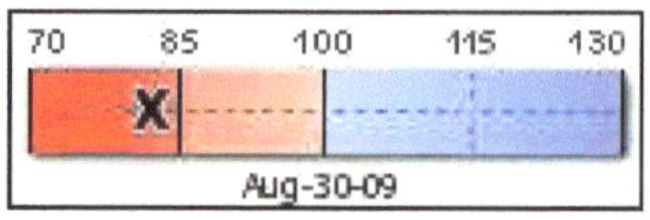

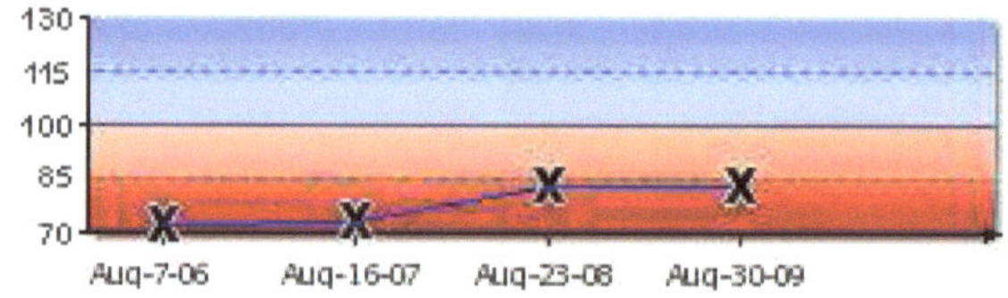

Executive Function: 102.2

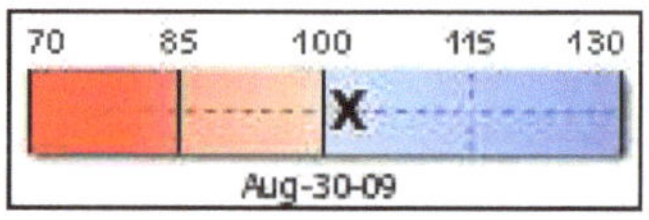

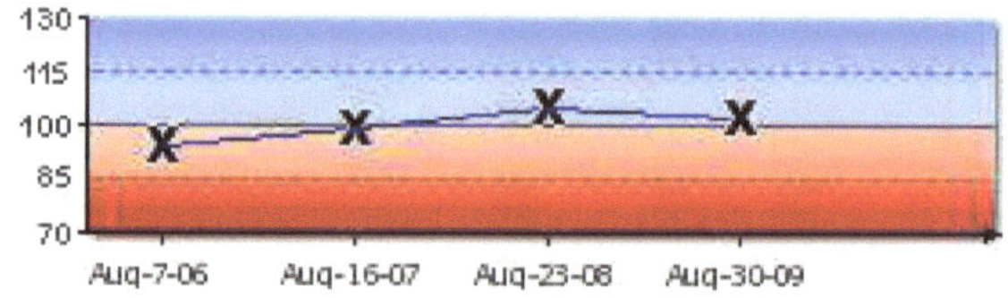

Attention: 97.4

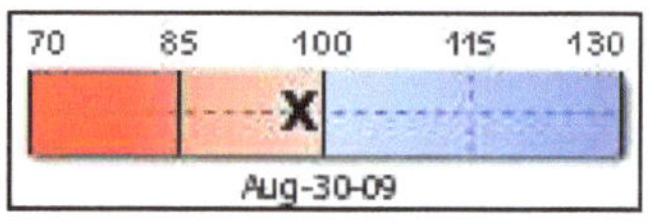

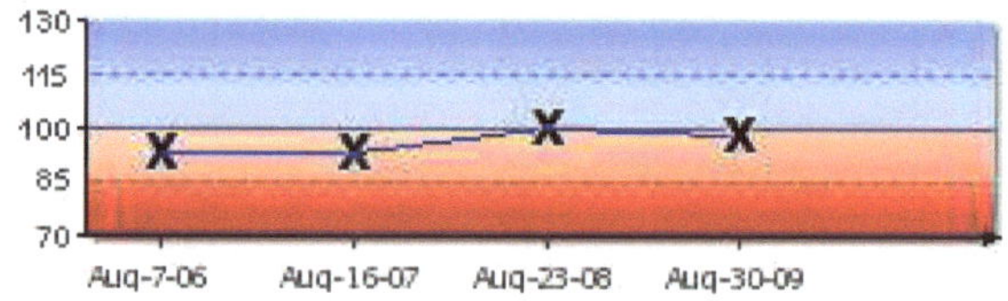

Information Processing Speed: 84.8

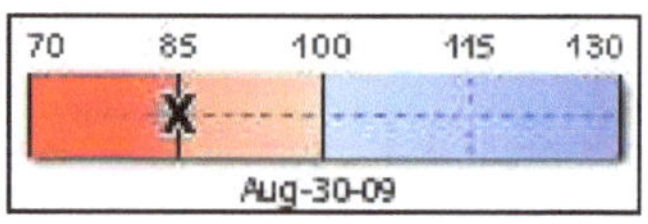

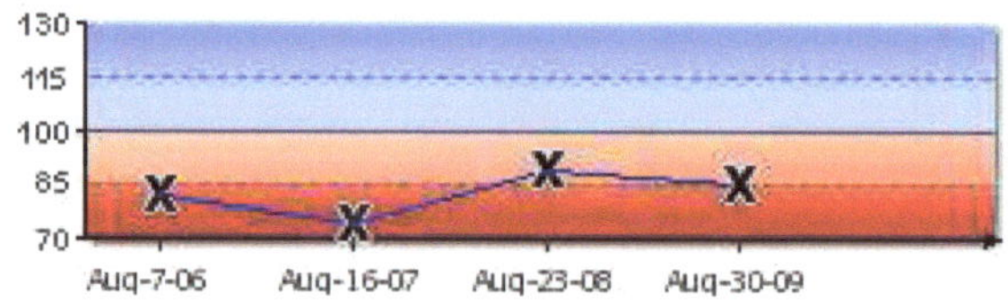

Visual Spatial: 97.1

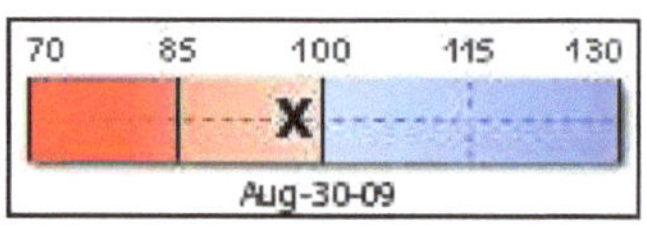

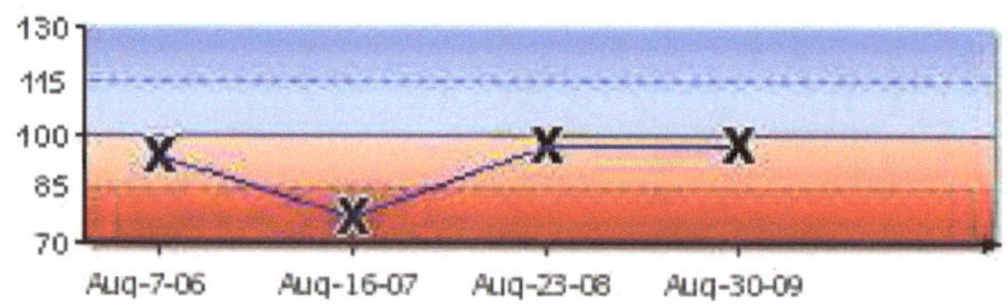

Verbal Function: 103

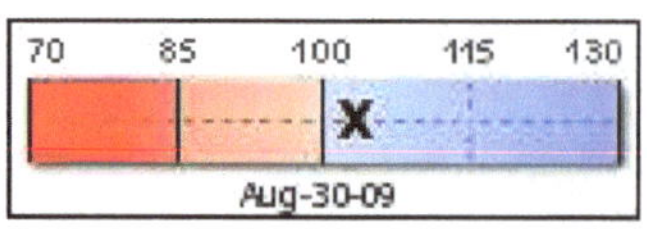

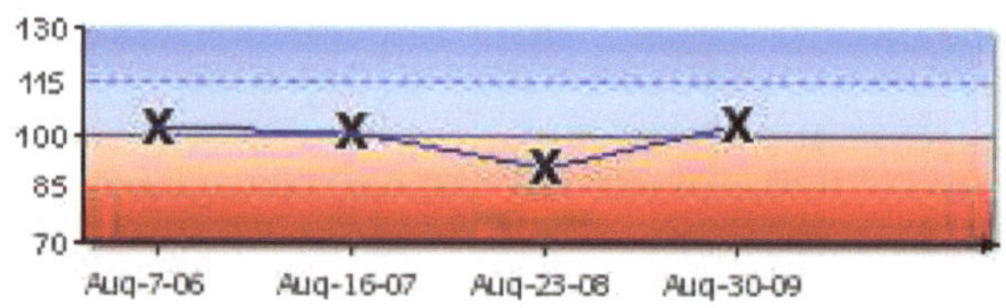

Motor Skills: 113.5

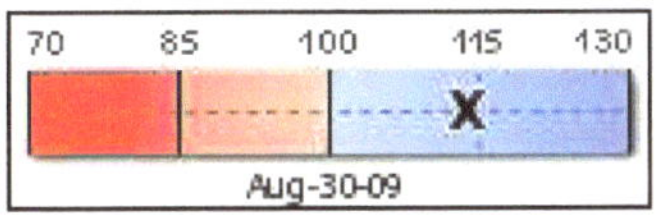

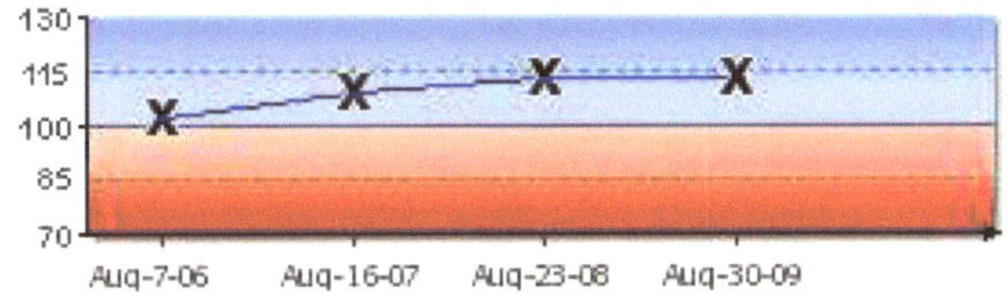

Index Score Legend

	Aug-7-06 11:13 AM	Aug-16-07 9:42 AM	Aug-23-08 10:03 AM	Aug-30-09 9:57 AM
Global Cognitive Score	**91**	**89.4**	**96.7**	**97.2**
Memory	**70.8**	**72.5**	**82**	**82**
Verbal Memory: Total Accuracy	64.0	64.0	62.8	64.9
Delayed Verbal Memory: Accuracy	61.8	78.8	74.8	74.8
Non-Verbal Memory: Total Accuracy	80.8	76.9	101.3	99.1
Delayed Non-Verbal Memory: Accuracy	76.7	70.4	89.1	89.1
Executive Function	**94**	**99**	**105.6**	**102.2**
Go-NoGo: Composite Score	86.2	101.4	106.6	105.9
Stroop Interference: Composite Score, Level 3	90.8	82.6	84.3	81.3
Catch Game: Total Score	105.1	113.1	125.9	119.4
Attention	**93.1**	**93.1**	**99.5**	**97.4**
Go-NoGo: Rsp Time	84.2	101.0	105.9	103.4
Go-NoGo: Rsp Time Std Dev	72.6	103.8	108.4	91.4
Stroop Interference: Rsp Time, Level 2	108.4	107.1	100.9	112.4
Staged Info Proc: Rsp Time, Level 1.2	98.6	78.2	97.4	100.9
Staged Info Proc: Accuracy, Level 2.3	101.5	75.3	84.9	79.1
Information Processing Speed	**81**	**73.5**	**88.5**	**84.8**
Staged Info Proc: Composite Score, Level 1.1	100.7	120.5	101.1	91.9
Staged Info Proc: Composite Score, Level 1.3	96.7	96.7	96.6	93.9
Staged Info Proc: Composite Score, Level 2.1	71.7	69.7	73.9	86.6
Staged Info Proc: Composite Score, Level 2.2	75.2	52.9	92.3	77.1
Visual Spatial	**94**	**76.4**	**97.1**	**97.1**
Visual Spatial Processing: Accuracy	94.0	76.4	97.1	97.1
Verbal Function	**102.6**	**101.4**	**91.1**	**103**
Verbal Function: Rhyming, Accuracy	102.6	101.4	91.1	103.0
Motor Skills	**101.6**	**109.5**	**113.2**	**113.5**
Finger Tapping: Inter-Tap Interval	102.2	105.4	107.6	109.9
Finger Tapping: Tap Interval Std Dev	95.7	112.4	110.7	110.7
Catch Game: Time to Make 1st Move	107.0	110.7	121.2	120.1

DI - Data Insufficient for a Score

'Composite Score' is computed from Accuracy and Response Time.
Rsp Time and Rsp Time Std Dev computed for correct responses.

Detailed Test Results

	Aug-7-06 11:13 AM		Aug-16-07 9:42 AM		Aug-23-08 10:03 AM		Aug-30-09 9:57 AM	
	NORM	RAW	NORM	RAW	NORM	RAW	NORM	RAW
COMPUTER ORIENTATION								

Mouse: Accuracy		100%		100%		100%		100%
Keyboard: Accuracy		100%		100%		100%		100%
Word Reading: Accuracy		100%		100%		100%		100%
Picture Identification: Accuracy		100%		100%		100%		75%
Color Discrimination: Accuracy		100%		100%		100%		100%

GO-NOGO RESPONSE INHIBITION	N	R	N	R	N	R	N	R
Accuracy	112.7	100%	107.6	97%	108.7	97%	113.2	100%
Response Time	84.2	577ms	101.0	461ms	105.9	471ms	103.4	491ms
Response Time Standard Deviation	72.6	257ms	103.8	105ms	108.4	98ms	91.4	195ms
Errors of Commission (max. 12)	114.8	0	106.4	1	107.2	1	109.2	0
Errors of Omission (max. 18)	105.1	0	105.1	0	107.7	0	107.7	0
Response Time for Errors of Commission	-	-	83.0	581ms	95.7	515ms	-	-

VERBAL MEMORY	N	R	N	R	N	R	N	R
Immediate Recognition								
Accuracy, Repetition 1	73.7	20%	80.1	30%	76.5	20%	82.8	30%
Accuracy, Repetition 2	68.4	30%	75.1	40%	65.6	20%	65.6	20%
Accuracy, Repetition 3	67.1	30%	61.0	20%	62.8	20%	62.8	20%
Accuracy, Repetition 4	66.5	30%	60.5	20%	63.0	20%	63.0	20%
Delayed Recognition								
Accuracy	61.8	10%	78.8	40%	74.8	30%	74.8	30%

NON-VERBAL MEMORY	N	R	N	R	N	R	N	R
Immediate Recognition								
Accuracy, Repetition 1	102.2	50%	84.9	25%	108.4	50%	87.9	25%
Accuracy, Repetition 2	78.1	25%	78.1	25%	96.8	50%	96.8	50%
Accuracy, Repetition 3	78.7	25%	78.7	25%	109.7	75%	109.7	75%
Accuracy, Repetition 4	77.2	25%	77.2	25%	93.2	50%	100.1	63%
Delayed Recognition								
Accuracy	76.7	25%	70.4	13%	89.1	38%	89.1	38%

PROBLEM SOLVING	N	R	N	R	N	R	N	R
Accuracy (Non-Verbal IQ)	90.6	36%	83.5	24%	88.5	28%	86.2	24%

STROOP INTERFERENCE	N	R	N	R	N	R	N	R
No Interference: Letter Color [1]								
Accuracy	95.6	90%	108.2	100%	109.6	100%	109.6	100%
Response Time	106.8	645ms	105.9	669ms	109.9	602ms	112.3	522ms
Response Time Standard Deviation	110.1	179ms	111.3	155ms	109.8	188ms	111.4	150ms
No Interference: Word Meaning [2]								
Accuracy	107.7	100%	107.7	100%	107.2	100%	107.2	100%
Response Time	108.4	528ms	107.1	551ms	100.9	711ms	112.4	524ms
Response Time Standard Deviation	105.3	160ms	104.9	168ms	91.4	375ms	111.5	97ms
Interference: Color vs. Meaning [3]								
Accuracy	89.5	40%	81.6	20%	78.1	20%	74.9	13%
Response Time	105.2	650ms	100.7	795ms	104.4	822ms	92.4	1231ms
Response Time Standard Deviation	108.8	150ms	106.2	211ms	109.7	230ms	109.2	243ms

FINGER TAPPING	N	R	N	R	N	R	N	R
Inter-Tap Interval	102.2	215ms	105.4	206ms	107.6	207ms	109.9	199ms
Tap Interval Standard Deviation	95.7	42ms	112.4	19ms	110.7	12ms	110.7	12ms

Catch Game	N	R	N	R	N	R	N	R
Time to Make 1st Move	107.0	676ms	110.7	627ms	121.2	557ms	120.1	572ms
Time to Make 1st Move Standard Deviation	114.1	134ms	112.4	146ms	117.1	129ms	120.8	99ms
Average Direction Changes Per Trial	114.2	0.10	110.7	0.15	114.0	0.15	114.0	0.15
Total Score (max. 1000)	105.1	649	113.1	760	125.9	840	119.4	749

Staged Information Processing Speed	N	R	N	R	N	R	N	R
SINGLE DIGIT								
Slow Speed [1.1]								
Accuracy	103.7	100%	103.7	100%	105.3	100%	88.1	90%
Response Time	102.8	755ms	116.9	622ms	102.2	761ms	99.6	789ms
Response Time Standard Deviation	109.4	144ms	122.6	66ms	113.9	109ms	109.0	146ms
Medium Speed [1.2]								
Accuracy	105.8	100%	73.1	90%	105.2	100%	105.2	100%
Response Time	98.6	668ms	78.2	800ms	97.4	720ms	100.9	687ms
Response Time Standard Deviation	88.8	224ms	85.8	238ms	80.4	290ms	89.1	240ms
Fast Speed [1.3]								
Accuracy	110.6	100%	110.6	100%	98.7	90%	85.8	80%
Response Time	86.8	675ms	86.4	677ms	100.8	700ms	105.8	654ms
Response Time Standard Deviation	73.9	223ms	90.3	165ms	77.7	324ms	109.4	131ms
TWO-DIGIT ARITHMETIC								
Slow Speed [2.1]								
Accuracy	41.2	60%	96.1	90%	69.2	60%	101.6	90%
Response Time	98.4	1356ms	44.3	2163ms	81.3	1803ms	76.9	1886ms
Response Time Standard Deviation	63.1	662ms	94.6	405ms	101.2	373ms	108.0	312ms
Medium Speed [2.2]								
Accuracy	96.1	90%	32.0	50%	111.6	100%	81.9	70%
Response Time	62.6	1476ms	69.3	1402ms	78.9	1439ms	74.2	1508ms
Response Time Standard Deviation	68.4	394ms	43.4	512ms	87.1	335ms	66.2	463ms
Fast Speed [2.3]								
Accuracy	101.5	60%	75.3	PP	84.9	30%	79.1	20%
Response Time	103.2	845ms	68.3	PP	81.7	1197ms	140.5	345ms
Response Time Standard Deviation	94.6	227ms	57.6	PP	119.5	75ms	98.7	250ms
THREE-DIGIT ARITHMETIC								
Slow Speed [3.1]								
Accuracy	DI	DI	55.2	30%	DI	DI	49.0	30%
Response Time	DI	DI	105.8	1577ms	DI	DI	126.6	1355ms
Response Time Standard Deviation	DI	DI	81.3	700ms	DI	DI	53.5	1135ms
Medium Speed [3.2]								
Accuracy	DI	DI	71.3	PP	DI	DI	75.2	PP
Response Time	DI	DI	73.9	PP	DI	DI	76.8	PP
Response Time Standard Deviation	DI	DI	73.7	PP	DI	DI	67.4	PP
Fast Speed [3.3]								
Accuracy	DI	DI	87.1	PP	DI	DI	87.4	PP
Response Time	DI	DI	84.1	PP	DI	DI	88.1	PP
Response Time Standard Deviation	DI	DI	83.3	PP	DI	DI	85.4	PP

Verbal Function	N	R	N	R	N	R	N	R
Rhyming, Accuracy	102.6	75%	101.4	73%	91.1	51%	103.0	76%
Matching, Accuracy	92.2	83%	100.4	90%	107.9	97%	89.2	77%

Visual Spatial Processing	N	R	N	R	N	R	N	R
Accuracy	94.0	44%	76.4	19%	97.1	38%	97.1	38%

NAB - Not Available for Battery Ordered
DI - Data Insufficient for a Score
FP - Failed Practice
PP - Poor Performance

Rsp Time and Rsp Time Std Dev computed for correct responses.

Interpretation of Performance Graphs

GENERAL

- Range of 1 standard deviation (SD) above and below the average score for a normative population of similar age and educational level is indicated on the graphs.
- Normative database ranges from ages 12-95 and contains 1,569 individuals as of March 2007.
- Scores are normalized to a standard scale (mean=100, SD=15).
- Scores outside the 70-130 range are plotted on the graphs as circles.
- Timeline charts are shown if the patient has had two or more testing sessions.
- Invalid scores do not appear on the timeline charts.
- Dates of invalid scores appear in parentheses.

GUIDE TO INTERPRETATION

- Sometimes, patients may score poorly on a given day due to factors that do not represent their general cognitive abilities (e.g. medications that make the patient drowsy, insufficient sleep, or an acute medical illness). If there is suspicion of such, the Mindstreams® testing should be repeated on a day when the patient is at his usual level of function.
- Observation of the change in test scores over time is often helpful in supporting or refuting diagnoses for suspected neurodegenerative disease.

CAVEATS

THIS REPORT CONTAINS DATA THAT MUST BE INTEGRATED BY THE REFERRING PHYSICIAN WITH THE OTHER CLINICAL DATA AVAILABLE FOR THIS PATIENT. CORRELATION WITH OTHER CLINICAL DATA IS REQUIRED TO DETERMINE THE CLINICAL DIAGNOSIS. APPLICATION OF THE DATA HEREIN, ULTIMATE DIAGNOSTIC DETERMINATIONS, AS WELL AS TREATMENT DECISIONS BASED ON THIS DATA ARE THE SOLE RESPONSIBILITY OF THE REFERRING PHYSICIAN.

PEOPLE DIFFER IN BASELINE COGNITIVE ABILITIES. THEREFORE, REPEATED TESTING IS IMPORTANT WHEN EVALUATING FOR COGNITIVE DECLINE.

GENERAL CAUTION IN INTERPRETING COGNITIVE DATA

Assessment scores for a given testing session may be below the normal range for a variety of reasons. Before concluding that the results signify pathology:

- Check for acute or chronic medications that may cause cognitive slowing;
- Check for co-morbid medical conditions that may be associated with cognitive dysfunction;
- Understand the baseline functional capacity of the patient. If the patient is of below-average intelligence, he is likely to perform below the normative range of the population even in the absence of new cognitive pathology.

DISCLAIMER

The information provided by NeuroTrax® on the basis of testing with Mindstreams® is of a general nature and is not medical advice, a diagnosis or treatment. The Mindstreams® assessment report does not constitute the practice of medicine or the provision of professional health care advice. The report provides your medical professional with information on how your performance relates to other people your age. NeuroTrax® is not responsible for any decisions made based on information in the report. Your medical professional has the sole responsibility for establishing diagnosis and suggesting appropriate treatment.

NeuroTrax® Mindstreams Clinical Summary

Patient Name: John Doe, ID 999999999 **Date of Testing:** Aug-30-09, 9:57 AM

TEST SUPERVISION

Supervisor Questionnaire

		1	2	3	4	5	
How difficult were the tests for the subject?	easy		✓				hard
Did the subject find the tests easy to use?	easy	✓					hard
Did the subject find the tests easy to understand?	easy	✓					hard
How well do you think the subject performed?	best		✓				poorest

Patient Cooperation

____

____

Comments

____

____

Name: ____________ **Signature:** ____________ **Date:** ____________

CLINICAL INTERPRETATION

Impression

____

____

____

Management Plan

____

____

____

Name: ____________ **Signature:** ____________ **Date:** ____________

Company	Psychology Software Tools, Inc.
Location	Sharpsburg, Pennsylvania, USA
Website	www.camci.us.com
Cognitive Test Product	CAMCI (Computer Assessment of Memory and Cognitive Impairment)
Test Features	
Testing Time	Self-paced, Average <25 minutes.
Testing Platform	The CAMCI system consists of the CAMCI software preinstalled on a medical grade tablet PC using a digitized stylus, which is tethered to the tablet, to allow input. No Internet connection is required.
Can be Administered by Office Staff?	Yes, with training. See Company End Notes Section for further detail.
Cognitive Domains Tested	Verbal memory, non-verbal memory, functional memory, incidental memory, attention, processing speed, executive function.
Test Primarily used for Detection of:	Mild Cognitive Impairment (MCI), Alzheimer's Disease, other dementia types
Test Validity and References	See Company End Notes Section for Test Validation References
Test Report Format	See sample report next page.
Pricing Information	CAMCI is currently being developed for clinical use, but has yet to receive FDA clearance to market. License options are expected to include annual subscriptions & per test fees.

CAMCI

Computer Assessment of Memory and Cognitive Impairment

MURPHY, John

ID **568132502**

Born **01-Aug-1938 (74y 0m)** *Gender* **Male** *Education* **18 year(s)** *Test Date* **10-Aug-2012**

INTERPRETATION:

This patient's score is **25.61**, which indicates cognitive function within the **impaired range**.

Score is based on selected measures shown on page 2 and is adjusted for age, education, and difficulty of each measure.

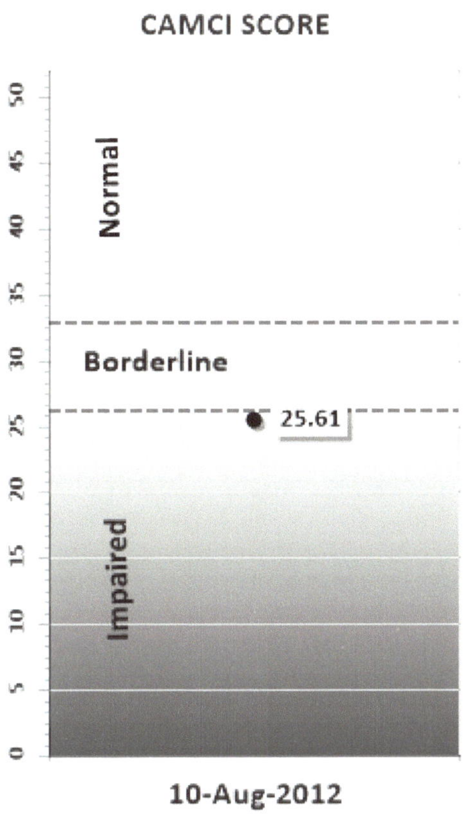

RECOMMENDATIONS:

- Review test results, including self-report, with patient and family to determine extent (if any) of everyday memory/cognitive problems. Assess functional status, review high level activities (e.g., managing finances, medications) and lower level activities (e.g., bathing, dressing).
- Initiate medical work-up to identify causes of cognitive impairment, for example as recommended by the American Geriatric Society guidelines*, including:
    - Conduct physical and neurologic examination, check esp. for focal weakness, gait impairment and parkinsonian features
    - Identify and treat illnesses such as hypertension and diabetes mellitus
    - Identify and treat reversible causes of cognitive impairment (e.g., B12 deficiency, thyroid disease, depression, sleep apnea)
    - Consider possible contribution of other medical factors to cognitive impairment, especially cerebrovascular and/or cardiovascular disease
    - Consider avoiding anticholinergic medications and limiting prn psychotropic medication
- Consider referral to specialist for comprehensive evaluation/treatment for possible neurodegenerative processes (e.g., brain imaging, neuropsychological work-up, identification of biomarkers for Alzheimer's disease, dementia medications)

SCREENING QUESTIONS (self-reported)			
SYMPTOMS		**ACTIVITIES**	
Depression	NO	Computer Use	YES
Anxiety	NO	ATM Use	YES
Alcohol Use	NO	Currently Drive	NO
Memory Decline	NO	Ever Driven	YES
Functional Decline	NO		
Orientation to Date:	Incorrect (Response: 7/10/2012)		

*Guide to Dementia Diagnosis and Treatment from the American Geriatrics Society, 2010 report. http://dementia.americangeriatrics.org/

Interpreting Healthcare Professional:

____

Review Date:

____

CAMCI
Computer Assessment of Memory and Cognitive Impairment

MURPHY, John

ID **568132502**

Born **01-Aug-1938 (74y 0m)** *Gender* **Male** *Education* **18 year(s)** *Test Date* **10-Aug-2012**

Task	Measure	Pass Threshold	Raw Score	
Simple Reaction Time	Number correct targets (out of 3)	≥ 3	3	
	Median reaction time (all responses) in msec.	**≤ 750**	**486**	
Digit Span Forward	**Maximum span (out of 6)**	**≥ 5**	**5**	
	Reaction time (first trial) in msec.	**≤ 5000**	**5218**	Out of range
Digit Span Reverse	**Maximum span (out of 5)**	**≥ 5**	**4**	Out of range
	Reaction time (first trial) in msec.	**≤ 3600**	**1591**	
Go/No Go	Rule 1 Number correct (out of 10)	≥ 8	10	
	Rule 2 Number correct (out of 10)	**≥ 9**	**10**	
Word Recall	**Number correct (out of 5)**	**≥ 3**	**3**	
	Number omissions (out of 5)	≤ 3	0	
Verbal Recognition	**Number correct (out of 6)**	**≥ 6**	**6**	
	Mean reaction time (all responses) in msec.	**≤ 5000**	**2863**	
Recurring Pictures	Number correct (out of 48)	≥ 38	44	
	Number correct first repeats (out of 8)	≥ 6	6	
	Signal detection statistic (d-prime)	**≥ 2.01**	**2.28**	
	Mean reaction time (correct first repeats) in msec.	**≤ 2750**	**1902**	
Virtual Environment	**Intersection accuracy (out of 18)**	**≥ 14**	**13**	Out of range
	Incidental recall number correct (out of 5)	**≥ 2**	**3**	
	Itemized recall number correct (out of 6)	**≥ 4**	**3**	Out of range
	ATM accuracy (out of 7)	≥ 5	7	

Measures in **bold** contribute to the overall CAMCI score on page 1

Out of range [flag]

Notes:

For additional information, please refer to the CAMCI Operator's Manual.

CAMCI is intended as a computerized assessment tool to contribute to the clinical assessment of cognitive function in older adults. CAMCI does not offer a medical diagnosis. The results of the CAMCI, when interpreted by a qualified healthcare professional, will assist in the identification of patients with suspected cognitive impairment for whom further evaluation may be appropriate. Refer to the Operator's Manual for a complete list of contraindications, warnings, and precautions associated with use of CAMCI.

Company	Screen, Inc.
Location	Seattle, Washington, USA
Website	www.screen-inc.com
Cognitive Test Product	CANS-MCI
Test Features	
Testing Time	30 minutes
Required Hardware	Touchscreen. Internet connection for report creation.
Can be Administered by Office Staff?	Yes, with brief training.
Cognitive Domains Tested	Immediate and Delayed Free and Cued Recall, Executive Functions, Word and Symbol Fluency.
Test Primarily Used for Detection of:	Mild Cognitive Impairment (MCI), Alzheimer's Disease, other dementia types
Test Validity and References	Significant test differences between normal controls and MCI subjects. See End Notes Section for further detail.
Test Report Format	MCI Probability Index Percentiles See sample report next page.
Pricing Information	Software (specific to each facility) free. Single session or longitudinal testing report fee per test. No volume or advance requirements. Contact Company for more detail.

SCREEN INC. PHYSICIAN REPORT

Computer-Administered Neuropsychological Screen for Mild Cognitive Impairment

Testing Facility
XXXXXXX Medicine

Report Recipient
email@doctors_office.net

PATIENT CODE
5431208

Sex: F
Age: 68.3

TEST LANGUAGE
English

SESSION DATES
7/23/2007 14:59
9/15/2008 10:55
12/3/2008 10:20
6/24/2009 11:34

FINDINGS

This person's overall cognitive function score is improved but still low compared to her initial performance and low normal for her age and education.

- The ***Memory*** factor score (acquisition and short-term retention) improved, but still indicated **low normal functioning**.
- The ***Fluency*** factor score (language and clock symbol fluency) declined, and indicated **low normal functioning**.
- The ***Executive Functions*** score (abilities to organize, respond quickly, and inhibit incorrect responses) improved, and indicated **normal functioning**.

Cognitive Scores Relative to Norm (z scores for similar Education Level)

Percentile	Memory Factor Score 7/23/07	9/15/08	12/3/08	6/24/09	Symbol Fluency Score 7/23/07	9/15/08	12/3/08	6/24/09	Executive Function Score 7/23/07	9/15/08	12/3/08	6/24/09
98th – top												
84th – 97th					1.13							
51st – 83rd	0.70	0.53				0.93	0.18		0.68	0.21		0.02
41st – 50th				-0.09							-0.20	
31st – 40th								-0.48				
17th – 30th			-0.88									
8th – 16th												
3rd – 7th												
1 – 2												
Bottom 1%												

Memory Factor Score — Symbol Fluency Score — Executive Function Score

PROBABILITY OF MCI

30-39 %

	7/23/07	9/15/08	12/3/08	6/24/09
< 10%	X			
10 – 19%		X		
20 – 29%				
30 – 39%				X
40 – 49%				
50 – 59%				
60 – 69%			X	
70 – 79%				
80 – 89%				
90 – 100%				

PREDICTION

Screen predicts that if this person were given a full neuropsychological evaluation, the likelihood of an MCI diagnosis would be moderate (less than 40%). This estimate is just within the limits for normal aging.

Mild Cognitive Impairment (MCI) refers to a transitional state between normal aging and a diagnosis of probable dementia.

OTHER FACTORS INFLUENCING PATIENT'S COGNITIVE STATUS

- **Depression Scale**: Depression can cause or be confused with cognitive impairments or subjective memory deficits. **This person only answered 4 of the 10 depression scale questions in the symptomatic direction, an improvement from the last test session (9 of 10, indicating a need for close attention to depression).**
- **Medications: Attention to the effects of medication interactions upon cognition is always advised.**

RECOMMENDATIONS

- **Follow-up testing (every 6 months) is now recommended.**
- **Further evaluation of emotional factors no longer appears necessary.**
- **A driving safety evaluation may be appropriate.**

Screen, Inc.
1-866-668-9038
3511 46th Avenue NE
Seattle, WA USA 98105
www.screen-inc.com

SCREEN INC. PHYSICIAN REPORT

Computer-Administered Neuropsychological Screen for Mild Cognitive Impairment

Testing Facility
XXXXXXX Medicine

Report Recipient
email@doctors_office.net

PATIENT CODE
5431208

Sex: F
Age: 68.3

TEST LANGUAGE
English

PERSONAL INFORMATION

- She reports 12 years of formal education.
- She has a history of head injury, a suspected risk factor, reporting more than 4 lifetime head injuries that caused unconsciousness.
- She has a history of exposure to solvents, reporting more than 20 years of occupational or other major exposure to solvents, a factor known to increase the risk of cognitive impairment.
- These test results must be interpreted in the context of pain medication use, since she reports using pain medication 5-6 times a week, and reports that the same amount of pain medication has less effect than it used to and she has to take more pills per day than the doctor directed.
- She may be deriving a preventive effect from more than 20 years of regular exercise.

DISCUSSION OF FINDINGS

- She shows a possible impairment in memory. This impairment in short-term memory might be apparent only to those closest to her and be evident in the form of a reduced ability to learn new information, keep track of appointments, or benefit from reminders.

- The possible impairment in fluency was significant with respect to identifying driving signs. This person reports driving within the last year and, therefore, received the driving-related Naming test (this test requires the selection of the correct 2-letter word beginning that matches each of 42 pictures). She was able to select the 2-letter word beginnings that matched 5 of the 14 driving signs and objects.

- The changes in cognitive functioning correlate highly with the changes in her depression scale scores.

This report has been produced by a live neuropsychology testing technician using scoring and test administration, not a licensed treatment provider. This report is neither intended nor approved for clinical diagnosis. Its purpose is to screen for the need to perform the professional tests which might be prescribed by the physician to determine specific medical diagnosis. The treating physician, not Screen, Inc., has sole responsibility for interpretation of this Report and any diagnoses and decisions based upon this Report.

Screen, Inc.
1-866-668-9038
3511 46th Avenue NE
Seattle, WA USA 98105
www.screen-inc.com

Mild Cognitive Impairment refers to a level of impairment in-between normal aging and the fully developed clinical features of dementia. These declines in memory and executive functions may occur up to 7 and3 years prior to Alzheimer's diagnosis, respectively. Since patients' cognitive functioning can change over time for many reasons, repeated (longitudinal testing is advised. The percentiles in the cognitive score tables correspond to standardized z-scores for people in the same education group, color-coded as follows: Greens: z better than 2:0; z between +1.01 and +2.00; z from 0.00(average) to +1.00. Yellow: z between –0.01 and –0.25, -0.26 to –0.50, -0.51 to –1.00, -1.01 to –1.50. Reds: -1.51 to –2.00; -2.01 to –3.00; less than –3.00.

ORGANIZATION	US DEPARTMENT OF DEFENSE
LOCATION	Washington DC, USA
WEBSITE	
COGNITIVE TEST PRODUCT	Defense Automated NeuroBehavioral Assessment (DANA)
TEST FEATURES	
TESTING TIME	5 -45 minutes, depending on testing level.
TESTING PLATFORM	Android mobile devices
CAN BE ADMINISTERED BY OFFICE STAFF?	Yes, by trained personnel.
COGNITIVE DOMAINS TESTED	Working Memory, Attention, Visual Memory, Psychomotor function, Psychological/Stress Metrics
TEST PRIMARILY USED FOR DETECTION OF:	Complex Traumatic Brain Injury (TBI) Symptoms, Post Traumatic Stress Disorder (PTSD) Symptoms
TEST VALIDITY AND REFERENCES	Currently in field validation trials.
TEST REPORT FORMAT	Currently in development.
PRICING INFORMATION	NA

PHYSICIAN USE CASE EXAMPLES

Use Case: Internal Medicine Practice

Dr. D practices internal medicine in rural New England. He is vigilant towards signs of memory loss and includes it as a topic on the Medical History forms that all patients complete. He also touches on memory loss in his clinical discussions with each elder patient. Whenever a concern is present, he schedules a follow-up appointment to complete a cognitive assessment using Medical Care Corporation's MCI Screen.

About one quarter of his patients over the age of 65 have some memory deficit, with a clear medical cause identified through a subsequent diagnostic work-up. The approximate distribution of clinical diagnoses in his practice is similar to published prevalence figures for the nation:

- Possible Alzheimer's disease 43%
- Cerebrovascular disease 36%
- Alcohol abuse 9%
- Traumatic brain injury 4%
- Depressive pseudodementia 3%
- Metabolic disorders 2%
- All others 3%

Interestingly, the majority of his patients screened for memory loss did not seek medical attention specifically for a memory concern, and would not likely have done so until the problem worsened. Dr. D's **early intervention is improving patient's lives and treating memory loss before the underlying problems cause further health problems**. Waiting until memory deficits are clearly present can degrade quality of life, and cause further health problems due to missed medication schedules and avoidable accidents.

PHYSICIAN USE CASE EXAMPLES (cont)

Use Case: Neurology Practice

A specialty practice with three neurologists in New York selected the NeuroTrax MindStreams cognitive screening tool as a method to provide objective testing for patients with memory complaints. MindStreams helps to differentiate normal age related cognitive performance from clinical mild cognitive impairment (MCI), and early signs of dementia.

Using a computerized cognitive test **allows the clinician to quietly evaluate** the patient's motor responses, area of struggles and attention while the patient is engaged with the MindStreams test.

Standardized reporting in MindStreams also helps explain the test results to the patient and family, improving patient and family satisfaction.

Use Case: Physician Group Practice

Summit Medical Group is a large primary care organization serving patients in eastern Tennessee. Summit has over 200 physicians on staff, and provides health care services through a number of offices, clinics, and labs. Summit chose Medinteract's COGselftest (CST) for a 6-month pilot program, before rolling out the CST to all Summit physicians.

The CST is a 10 minute computerized test that screens all six cognitive domains, which is critical to accurately detect various forms and degrees of impaired cognition. The CST can be performed in the physician's office, and is reimbursable by Medicare.

The test provides an objective cognitive score **that can be tracked over time** on repeat tests, which can assist physicians in **identifying serious declines** in cognitive health.

REPORT END NOTES

1. World Development Indicators Database, World Bank, 1 July 2011

2. Hurd MD, Martorell P, Delavande A, Mullen KJ, Langa KM. Monetary costs of dementia in the United States. N Engl J Med. 2013 Apr 4;368(14):1326-34. PubMed PMID: 23550670

3. Bateman RJ, et al, Dominantly Inherited Alzheimer Network. Clinical and biomarker changes indominantly inherited Alzheimer's disease. N Engl J Med. 2012 Aug 30;367(9):795-804.

4. World Alzheimer Report 2010, Alzheimer's Disease International (ADI) www.alz.co.uk/research/files/WorldAlzheimerReport2010.pdf

5. Faul M, Xu L, Wald MM, Coronado VG. Traumatic brain injury in the United States: emergency department visits, hospitalizations, and deaths. Atlanta (GA): Centers for Disease Control and Prevention, National Center for Injury Prevention and Control; 2010.

6. Adamson, David M., et al, Invisible Wounds of War: Psychological and Cognitive Injuries, Their Consequences, and Services to Assist Recovery. Santa Monica, CA: RAND Corporation, 2008. http://www.rand.org/pubs/monographs/MG720.

7. Perou R, Bitsko, et al, Division of Human Development and Disability, National Center on Birth Defects and Developmental Disabilities, CDC, Atlanta, Georgia (2013). Mental health surveillance among children - United States, 2005-2011. Morbidity and mortality weekly report. Surveillance summaries (Washington, D.C. : 2002), 62 (2), 1-35 PMID: 23677130

COMPANY END NOTES

BRAINFX
PRODUCT: BRAINFX
PRIMARY USE: CONCUSSION & COMPLEX TBI ASSESSMENT

Test Validation Studies - In Process

York University: Sergio, L., Gage, W. Brain Function: Comparing healthy individuals to individuals who have a history of concussion or brain injury using a new tablet-based assessment.

University of Toronto: Reed, N., Mihailidas, A. Performance comparison of athletes on baseline testing versus repeat testing post-concussion using a neurofunctional tablet based assessment tool.

Test-Retest Reliability

Validation studies in process

Normative Data Sample Size

Validation studies in process

Alternate Forms (for test battery)

None reported.

Brain Resource
Product: WebNeuro
Primary Use: Depression screening, other neuropsychiatric disorders.

Test Validation References

Silverstein SM, Berten S, Olson P, Paul R, Willams LM, Cooper N, Gordon E. Development and validation of a World-Wide-Web-based neurocognitive assessment battery: WebNeuro. Behav Res Methods. 2007 Nov;39(4):940-9.

Mathersul D, Palmer DM, Gur RC, Gur RE, Cooper N, Gordon E, Williams LM. Explicit identification and implicit recognition of facial emotions: II. Core domains and relationships with general cognition. J Clin Exp Neuropsychol. 2009 Apr;31(3):278-91.

Williams LM, Mathersul D, Palmer DM, Gur RC, Gur RE, Gordon E. Explicit identification and implicit recognition of facial emotions: I. Age effects in males and females across 10 decades. J Clin Exp Neuropsychol. 2009 Apr;31(3):257-77.

Test-Retest Reliability

None reported.

Normative Data Sample Size

n>400 (age >50)

Alternate Forms (for test battery)

None reported.

Test Validation References

Corbett BA, Constantine LJ. Autism and attention deficit hyperactivity disorder: assessing attention and response control with the integrated visual and auditory continuous performance test. Child Neuropsychol. 2006 Aug;12(4-5):335-48. PubMed PMID: 16911977

Hagelthorn KM, Hiemenz JR, Pillion JP, Mahone EM. Age and task parameters in continuous performance tests for preschoolers. Percept Mot Skills. 2003 Jun;96(3 Pt 1):975-89. PubMed PMID: 12831279.

Tinius TP. The intermediate visual and auditory continuous performance test as a neuropsychological measure. Arch Clin Neuropsychol. 2003 Mar;18(2):199-214. PubMed PMID: 14591471

Xiong Z, Shi S, Xu H. A controlled study of the effectiveness of EEG biofeedback training on-children with attention deficit hyperactivity disorder. J Huazhong Univ Sci Technolog Med Sci. 2005;25(3):368-70. PubMed PMID: 16201300

Test-Retest Reliability

None reported.

Normative Data Sample Size

N=1700, ages 6-96

Alternate Forms (for test battery)

None reported.

Test Validation References

Blackwell AD, Sahakian BJ, Vesey R, Semple JM, Robbins TW, Hodges JR. (2004). Detecting dementia: novel neuropsychological markers of preclinical Alzheimer's disease. Dement Geriatr Cogn Disord. 17(1-2):428

Chandler J, Marsico M, Harper-Mozley L, Vogt R, Peng Y, Lesk V & DeJager, C (2008). Cognitive assessment: Discrimination of impairment and detection of decline in Alzheimer's disease and mild cognitive impairment. Alzheimer's and Dementia. 4(4):T551-T552.

de Rover M, et al,. (2011). Hippocampal dysfunction in patients with mild cognitive impairment: a functional neuroimaging study of a visuospatial paired associates learning task. Neuropsychologia. 49(7):2060-70.

Fowler KS, Saling MM, Conway EL, Semple JM, Louis WJ. (2002). Paired associate performance in the early detection of DAT. J Int Neuropsychol Soc.8(1):58-71

Mitchell J, Arnold R, Dawson K, Nestor PJ, Hodges JR. (2009). Outcome in subgroups of mild cognitive impairment (MCI) is highly predictable using a simple algorithm. Journal of Neurology. 256(9):1500-9.

Saunders NL, Summers MJ. (2011). Longitudinal deficits to attention, executive, and working memory in subtypes of mild cognitive impairment. Neuropsychology. 25(2):237-48.

Test-Retest Reliability

None reported

Normative Data Sample Size

n=787 (55-80)

Alternate Forms (for test battery)

None reported.

CNS Vital Signs

Product: CNS Vital Signs

Primary Use: MCI, Alzheimer's Disease, other dementia types

Test Validation References
Summary: CNS Vital Signs was developed for use in both primary care and specialist practices. Gualtieri CT, Johnson LG. Neurocognitive testing supports a broader concept of mild cognitive impairment. Am J Alzheimers Dis Other Demen 2005;20:359–366. Gualtieri CT, Johnson LG. Reliability and validity of a computerized neurocognitive test battery,CNS Vital Signs. Arch Clin Neuropsychol 2006;21:623–643.
Test-Retest Reliability
.56 to .90 after 1-282 days
Normative Data Sample Size
n=233 (50+)
Alternate Forms (for test battery)
Unlimited

CogState
Product: COGNIGRAM
Primary Use: MCI, Alzheimer's Disease, other dementia types

Test Validation References

Lim YY, Ellis KA, Harrington K, Ames D, Martins RN, Masters CL, et al. Use of the CogState Brief Battery in the assessment of Alzheimer's disease related cognitive impairment in the Australian Imaging, Biomarkers and Lifestyle (AIBL) study. J Clin Exp.Neuropsychol. 2012;34(4):345-58.

Maruff P, Thomas E, Cysique L, Brew B, Collie A, Snyder P, et al. Validity of the CogState brief battery: relationship to standardized tests and sensitivity to cognitive impairment in mild traumatic brain injury, schizophrenia, and AIDS dementia complex. Arch.Clin Neuropsychol. 2009;24(2):165-78.

Darby DG, Brodtmann A, Pietrzak RH, Fredrickson J, Woodward M, Villemagne VL, et al. Episodic memory decline predicts cortical amyloid status in community-dwelling older adults. J Alzheimers.Dis 2011;27(3):627-37.

Makdissi M, Darby D, Maruff P, Ugoni A, Brukner P, McCrory PR. Natural history of concussion in sport: markers of severity and implications for management. Am J Sports Med 2010;38(3):464-71.

Test-Retest Reliability

None reported

Normative Data Sample Size

None reported

Alternate Forms (for test battery)

None reported

HeadMinder
Product: CST
Primary Use: MCI, Alzheimer's Disease, other dementia types

Test Validation References

Summary: HeadMinder CST was developed for use in both primary care and specialist practices.

Erlanger DM, Kaushik T, Broshek D, Freemand J, Feldman D, Festa J. Development and validations of a web-based screening tool for monitoring cognitive status. J Head Trauma Rehab 2002;17:458–476.

Lichtenberg PA, Johnson AS, Erlanger DM, Kaushik T, Maddens ME, Imam K, et al. Enhancing cognitive screening in geriatric care: Use of an internet-based system. Int J Healthcare Inf Sys Informatics 2006;1:47–57.

Test-Retest Reliability

.68 to .94

Normative Data Sample Size

n=105 (65+)

Alternate Forms (for test battery)

Yes, multiple alternate forms.

IMPACT APPLICATIONS, INC.
PRODUCT: IMPACT
PRIMARY USE: CONCUSSION SYMPTOMS

Test Validation References

Lovell MR, Iverson GL, Collins MW, Podell K, Johnston KM, Pardini D, Pardini J, Norwig J, Maroon JC. Measurement of symptoms following sports-related concussion: reliability and normative data for the post-concussion scale. Appl Neuropsychol. 2006;13(3):166-74. PubMed PMID: 17361669.

Iverson GL, Lovell MR, Collins MW. Validity of ImPACT for measuring processing speed following sports-related concussion. J Clin Exp Neuropsychol. 2005 Aug;27(6):683-9. PubMed PMID: 16019644.

Iverson GL, Lovell MR, Collins MW. Interpreting change on ImPACT following sport concussion. Clin Neuropsychol. 2003 Nov;17(4):460-7. PubMed PMID: 15168911.

Schatz P, Pardini JE, Lovell MR, Collins MW, Podell K. Sensitivity and specificity of the ImPACT Test Battery for concussion in athletes. Arch Clin Neuropsychol. 2006 Jan;21(1):91-9. Epub 2005 Sep 6. PubMed PMID: 16143492.

Zuckerman SL, Lee YM, Odom MJ, Solomon GS, Forbes JA, Sills AK. Recovery from sports-related concussion: Days to return to neurocognitive baseline in adolescents versus young adults. Surg Neurol Int. 2012;3:130. Epub 2012 Oct 27. PubMed PMID: 23227435

Test-Retest Reliability

.15 - .39

Normative Data Sample Size

>1,000 ages 11+

Alternate Forms (for test battery)

100+

Medical Care Corp.
Product: MCI-Screen
Primary Use: MCI, Alzheimer's Disease, other dementia types

Test Validation References

Summary: MCI-Screen was developed for use in both primary care and specialist practices.

Shankle WR, Mangrola T, Chan T, Hara J. Development and validation of the Memory Performance Index: Reducing measurement error in recall tests. Alzheimer's & Dementia 5 (2009) 295–306.

Cohen M. Improved Mental Screening Can Cut Claim Costs. A new look at dementia claims by screened policyholders. National Underwriter Life & Health. Nov. 2009: 1-2.

Pooley. J.P., Lee, M.D., & Shankle. W.R. (in press, 2011). Understanding Alzheimer's using memory models and hierarchical Bayesian analysis. Journal of Mathematical Psychology.

Trenkle DL, Shankle WR, Azen SP. Detecting cognitive impairment in primary care: Performance assessment of three screening instruments. J Alzheimer's Dis 2007;11:323–335.

Shankle WR, Romney AK, Hara J, Fortier D, Dick MB, Chen JM, et al. Methods to improve the detection of mild cognitive impairment. PNAS 2005;102:4919–4924.

Test-Retest Reliability

.83 after 90 days

Normative Data Sample Size

n=471 (50+)

Alternate Forms (for test battery)

Yes, multiple alternate forms

MEDINTERACT

PRODUCT: COGSELFTEST

PRIMARY USE: MCI, ALZHEIMER'S DISEASE, OTHER DEMENTIA TYPES

Test Validation References

Summary: The MedInteract Computer Self Test is a new web-based screening tool for MCI and early AD.

Dougherty JH Jr, Cannon RL, Nicholas CR, Hall L, Hare F, Carr E, Dougherty A, Janowitz J, Arunthamakun J. The computerized self test (CST): an interactive, internet accessible cognitive screening test for dementia. J Alzheimers Dis. 2010;20(1):185-95

Monica K Crane, Rex L Cannon, Tarah Kuhn, Sadie Marnon, Andrew Dougherty, John H Dougherty Jr Computer Self-Test (CST) generated cognitive patterns: distinguishing among frontotemporal dementia, Alzheimer's disease and healthy older adults. Academic poster, American Academy of Neurology 2011 annual meeting.

Test-Retest Reliability

.80 after six weeks

Normative Data Sample Size

n=247 (50+)

Alternate Forms (for test battery)

None reported.

Test Validation References

Summary: MindStreams® is designed primarily for the identification and longitudinal tracking of elderly individuals at risk for MCI and early AD.

NeuroTrax has developed a 30-minute battery assessing memory, executive function, attention, and visual spatial function, the domains most relevant for MCI on the basis of the Dwolatzky et al. (2003) validity study and other literature (Chen et al., 2000; Reid et al., 1996; Mapstone et al., 2003; Kawas et al., 2003). Called the 'MCI Assessment Battery' (MAB; formerly the 'Early Dementia Battery'), discriminant validity for this battery was compared with that of the original 'Global Assessment Battery' (GAB; Dwolatzky et al., 2003) in a 2005 *Current Alzheimer Research* paper (Doniger et al., 2005). Discriminant validity for a measure of overall MAB performance was compared with that of an overall measure of GAB performance in 161 elderly participants from four centers. AUC from ROC analysis was comparable between MAB and GAB measures for discriminating dementia from non-dementia (GAB: 0.89, $p<0.001$; MAB: 0.89, $p<0.001$) and cognitively healthy from non-cognitively healthy (GAB: 0.81, $p<0.001$; MAB: 0.82, $p<0.001$), key clinical determinations for suggesting a diagnosis of MCI (i.e., not demented but not cognitively healthy). Moreover, both MAB and GAB measures discriminated well among cognitively healthy, MCI, and mild dementia groups ($p<0.001$).

Chen P, Ratcliff G, Belle SH, Cauley JA, DeKosky ST, Ganguli M. Cognitive tests that best discriminate between presymptomatic AD and those who remain nondemented. Neurology 2000;55:1847-53.

Doniger GM, Dwolatzky T, Zucker DM, Chertkow H, Crystal H, Schweiger A, Simon ES. Computerized cognitive testing battery identifies MCI and mild dementia even in the presence of depressive symptoms. Am J Alzheimers Dis Other Demen 2006;21:28-36.

Doniger GM, Simon DR, Dwolatzky T, Tanne D, Goldstein FC, Simon ES. Relevance of computerized cognitive assessment to functional disability in a mildly impaired elderly cohort. J Am Geriatr Soc 2009;57:S194.

Doniger GM, Simon ES, Schweiger A. Adjustment of cognitive scores with a co-normed estimate of premorbid intelligence: Implementation using Mindstreams computerized testing. Appl Neuropsychol 2008;15:250-63.

Doniger GM, Zucker DM, Schweiger A, Dwolatzky T, Simon ES. Towards practical cognitive assessment for detection of early dementia: A 30-minute computerized battery discriminates as well as longer testing. Curr Alzheimer Res 2005;2:117-24.

Dwolatzky T, Whitehead V, Doniger GM, Simon ES, Schweiger A, Jaffe D, Chertkow H. Validity of a novel computerized cognitive battery for mild cognitive impairment. BMC Geriatr 2003;3:4.

Fillit HM, Simon ES, Doniger GM, Cummings JL. Practicality of a computerized system for cognitive assessment in the elderly. Alzheimers Dement 2008;4:14-21.

Goldstein FC, Dwolatzky T, Doniger GM, Levey AI, Lah JJ, Simon ES. Computerized assessment reveals common deficits in multinational MCI cohort. Alzheimers Dement 2005;1:S18.

Kawas CH, Corrada MM, Brookmeyer R, Morrison A, Resnick SM, Zonderman AB, et al. Visual memory predicts Alzheimer's disease more than a decade before diagnosis. Neurology 2003;60:1089-93.

Mapstone M, Steffenella TM, Duffy CJ. A visuospatial variant of mild cognitive impairment: Getting lost between aging and AD. Neurology 2003;60:802-808.

Reid W, Broe G, Creasey H, Grayson D, McCusker E, Bennett H, et al. Age at onset and pattern of neuropsychological impairment in mild early-stage Alzheimer disease. A study of a community-based population. Arch Neurol 1996;53:1056-61.

Simon E, Doniger G. Idiopathic elderly fallers have a distinct cognitive profile from amnestic MCI, early Alzheimer's disease, and Parkinson's disease: A review of studies using Mindstreams computerized cognitive assessment. [Symposium: Computerized testing and assessment II: Detection and diagnosis of mild cognitive impairment (MCI), dementia and cognitive impairment in older adults. An update for clinical neuropsychologists.] J Int Neuropsychol Soc 2008;14(S1):125.

Simon ES, Goldstein FC, Dwolatzky T, Levey AI, Lah JJ, Doniger GM. A prospective study of cognitive performance in amnestic MCI using comprehensive computerized assessment. Alzheimers Dement 2006;2:S288.

Simon ES, Goldstein FC, Lah JJ, Doniger GM, Levey AI, Dwolatzky T. Computerized cognitive assessment predicts conversion to dementia within two years: Interim analysis of a prospective study of MCI. Int Conf Prev Dement (June 9-12, Washington, DC) 2007, Abst HT-523.

Test-Retest Reliability

Equivalence for two alternate forms (correlation coefficients: Memory $r = 0.84$, Executive Function $r = 0.80$, Visual Spatial $r = 0.64$, Verbal $r = 0.40$, Attention $r = 0.79$, Information Processing $r = 0.68$, Motor Skills $r = 0.80$) was demonstrated in a cohort of 57 healthy middle-age volunteers retested at a median interval of 4.84 weeks (Schweiger et al., 2003). Equivalence for all three alternate forms (correlation coefficients: Memory $0.80 \leq r \leq 0.84$, Executive Function $0.62 \leq r \leq 0.73$, Visual Spatial $0.68 \leq r \leq 0.83$, Verbal $0.51 \leq r \leq 0.63$, Attention $0.67 \leq r \leq 0.78$, Information Processing $0.73 \leq r \leq 0.85$, Motor Skills $0.62 \leq r \leq 0.77$) was demonstrated in a 2005 US Navy report stating that "the measures appear to demonstrate acceptable test-retest reliability coefficients as well as the alternate form reliability coefficients." The report further stated that the equivalence "reduces the learning effect that can occur after repeated exposures, it allows for increased accuracy in interpreting results, and it decreases the possibility of underestimating an actual impairment." (Melton, 2005)

Normative Data Sample Size

n=805 (age >50); *n*=1569, (age >8)

Alternate Forms (for entire test battery)

Yes; 3 alternate forms

Psychology Software Tools
Product: CAMCI (Computer Assessment of Memory and Cognitive Impairment)
Primary Use: MCI, Alzheimer's Disease, other dementia types

Test Validation References

Summary: CAMCI is a new tablet based screening tool for MCI and early AD.

Saxton J, Morrow L, Eschman A, Archer G, Luther J, Zuccolotto A. Computer Assessment of Mild Cognitive Impairment. Postgraduate Medicine. 2009 Mar; 121(2):177-85. PMID: 19332976

Nieto ML, Albert SM, Morrow LA, Saxton J. Cognitive status and physical function in older african americans. Journal of the American Geriatrics Society. 2008; 56(11):2014–2019. PMID: 18811612

Tierney MC, Lermer MA. Computerized cognitive assessment in primary care to identify patients with suspected cognitive impairment. Journal of Alzheimers Disesae. 2010; 20(3):823-32. PMID: 20413868

Snyder PJ, Jackson CE, Petersen RC, Khachaturian AS, Kaye J, Albert M, Weintraub S. Assessment of cognition in mild cognitive impairment: The Campaign to Prevent Alzheimer's Disease by 2020 comparative survey. Alzheimers & Dementia. 2011; 7(3):338-55. PMID: 21575877

Becker, JT, Dew, MA, Aizenstein, HJ, Lopez, OL, Morrow, L, Saxton, J. Concurrent validity of a computer-based cognitive screening tool for use in adults with HIV disease. AIDS Patient Care STDS 2011, Jun; 25(6): 3651-7. PMID: 21545295

Test-Retest Reliability

.63, after 4 weeks

Normative Data Sample Size

537 (60-93 years)

Alternate Forms (for test battery)

Currently being validated.

Test Validation References

Summary: CANS-MCI was developed for use in both primary care and specialist practices.

Jane B. Tornatore, PhD Emory Hill, PhD Jo Anne Laboff, MSW Self-Administered Screening for Mild Cognitive Impairment: Validation of a Computerized Test Battery. Journal of Neuropsychiatry and Clinical Neurosciences, Volume 17, No. 1, 98-105, Winter, 2005.

Jane B. Tornatore, PhD, Emory Hill, PhD, Jo A. Laboff, MSW, Brian Fogel Preliminary Screening for Mild Cognitive Impairment (MCI): Using the CANS-MCI in Primary Care to Determine Need for Imaging. 9th International Conference on Alzheimer's Disease, Philadelphia, PA, July, 2004.

Jane B. Tornatore, PhD, Emory Hill, PhD, Jo A. Laboff, MSW, Brian Fogel One year Follow-Up Analyses of Scoring Algorithms for a Mild Cognitive Impairment (MCI) Screen: The CANS-MCI Study. Alzheimer's Association International Conference on Prevention of Dementia: Early Diagnosis and Intervention, Washington, DC, June, 2005.

Celeste de Jager and Samrah Ali The Utility and Sensitivity of Traditional and Novel Cognitive Screening Tools for MCI. 2009. Unpublished.

Wild K, Howieson D, Webbe F, Seelye A, Kaye J. Status of computerized cognitive testing in aging: a systematic review. Alzheimers Dementia. 2008; 4(6):428–437. Each test battery was rated on the availability of normative data, level of evidence for test validity & reliability, comprehensiveness and usability.

Test-Retest Reliability

.65 -.88 after one month

Normative Data Sample Size

n=233 (50+)

Alternate Forms (for test battery)

None reported.

Test Validation Studies - In Process

Henry M. Jackson Foundation for the Advancement of Military Medicine. PI: Jack Tsao, US Department of Defense. Comparison of the DANA to the ANAM in the Evaluation of Cognitive Changes After Concussion

Test-Retest Reliability

Validation studies in process

Normative Data Sample Size

Validation studies in process

Alternate Forms (for test battery)

None reported

www.ingramcontent.com/pod-product-compliance
Lightning Source LLC
LaVergne TN
LVHW072013300926
849160LV00002B/10